Shanmughavel Piramanayagam

Studies on Human alpha 7 Nicotinic Acetylcholine receptor

Shanmughavel Piramanayagam

Studies on Human alpha 7 Nicotinic Acetylcholine receptor

Structural Insight Studies on Human alpha 7 Nicotinic Receptor in response to Neurotoxins and Neurotransmitters

VDM Verlag Dr. Müller

Impressum/Imprint (nur für Deutschland/ only for Germany)
Bibliografische Information der Deutschen Nationalbibliothek: Die Deutsche Nationalbibliothek verzeichnet diese Publikation in der Deutschen Nationalbibliografie; detaillierte bibliografische Daten sind im Internet über http://dnb.d-nb.de abrufbar.

Coverbild: www.purestockx.com

Verlag: VDM Verlag Dr. Müller Aktiengesellschaft & Co. KG
Dudweiler Landstr. 99, 66123 Saarbrücken, Deutschland
Telefon +49 681 9100-698, Telefax +49 681 9100-988, Email: info@vdm-verlag.de
Zugl.: Coimbatore, Bharathiar University, 2009

Herstellung in Deutschland:
Schaltungsdienst Lange o.H.G., Berlin
Books on Demand GmbH, Norderstedt
Reha GmbH, Saarbrücken
Amazon Distribution GmbH, Leipzig
ISBN: 978-3-639-18807-3

Imprint (only for USA, GB)
Bibliographic information published by the Deutsche Nationalbibliothek: The Deutsche Nationalbibliothek lists this publication in the Deutsche Nationalbibliografie; detailed bibliographic data are available in the Internet at http://dnb.d-nb.de .

Cover image: www.purestockx.com

Publisher:
VDM Verlag Dr. Müller Aktiengesellschaft & Co. KG
Dudweiler Landstr. 99, 66123 Saarbrücken, Germany
Phone +49 681 9100-698, Fax +49 681 9100-988, Email: info@vdm-publishing.com

Printed in the U.S.A.
Printed in the U.K. by (see last page)
ISBN: 978-3-639-18807-3

A STRUCTURAL INSIGHT STUDIES ON HUMAN NEURONAL α_7 NICOTINIC ACETYLCHOLINE RECEPTOR IN RESPONSE TO NEUROTOXINS AND NEUROTRANSMITTERS

M.Parthiban
Dr.P.Shanmughavel Ph.D.,D.Sc.

DEPARTMENT OF BIOINFORMATICS
BHARATHIAR UNIVERSITY
COIMBATORE - 640 046
INDIA

CONTENTS

A Structural insight studies on Human neuronal α_7 Nicotinic Acetylcholine Receptor (α_7nAChR) in Response to Neurotoxins and Neurotransmitters.

Acetylcholine receptors (AChR) in the mammalian Central Nervous System (CNS) can be divided into muscarinic (mAChR) and nicotinic (nAChR) subtypes based on the ability of the natural alkaloids, muscarine and nicotine, to mimic the effects of acetylcholine (ACh) as a neurotransmitter. The nicotinic Acetylcholine Receptor (nAChR) is the major class of neurotransmitter receptors that is present in the CNS and mainly involved in many neurodegenerative conditions such as Schizophrenia, Alzheimer's and Parkinson's diseases. The nicotinic AChRs are superfamily of Ligand-Gated Ion Channels (LGICs) that form pores in cells, plasma membranes, mediating fast signal transmission at synaptic gorge (Itier and Bertrand 2001). The neuronal nicotinic AChRs are located at synapses between neurons, such as the CNS where they are involved in cognitive function, learning, memory, arousal, motor control and analgesia [Fig. 1].

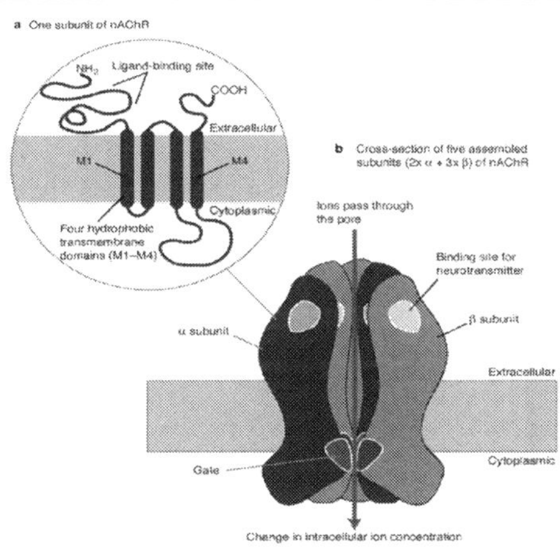

Figure 1: Structure of Nicotnic Acetylcholine Receptor

This superfamily of pentameric Ligand-Gated Ion Channels (LGICs), including nAChR, 5-HT$_3$, GABA$_{A,C}$ and glycine receptors, mediates chemical synaptic transmission. All of these LGICs form homo or hetero-pentamers of related subunits, implying a common evolutionary origin. Each subunit is divided into an N-terminal or Ligand-Binding Domain (LBD), a transmembrane and an intracellular region. The LBDs, which are around 210 amino-acid residues long, contain ligand-binding sites for agonists and competitive antagonists. Binding of an agonist induces rapid opening of the transmembrane ion channel, leading to a change in membrane potential. The signal transmission mechanism is explained by allosteric interactions between subunits, involving numerous conformational transitions (Hogg and Bertrand 2007).

The binding of neurotransmitters like acetylcholine to nAChRs brings about their channel activation. When two molecules of acetylcholine bind to nAChR, a conformational change occurs in the receptor, resulting in the formation of an ion pore (Karlin 2002). At the neuromuscular junction, the opening of a pore produces a rapid increase in the cellular permeability of sodium and calcium ions, resulting in the depolarisation and excitation of the muscle cell, thereby producing a muscular contraction. The activation of neuronal nicotinic AChRs also causes the movement of cations through the opening of an ion channel, with the influx of calcium ions affects the release of neurotransmitters. Nicotinic AChRs on a postganglionic neuron are responsible for the initial fast depolarisation of that neuron. The binding of nicotine can activate nAChRs, modifying the neurons in two ways: the depolarisation of the membrane through the movement of cations results in an excitation of the neuron, while the influx of calcium acts through intracellular cascades affect the regulation of certain genes and the release of neurotransmitters [Fig. 2].

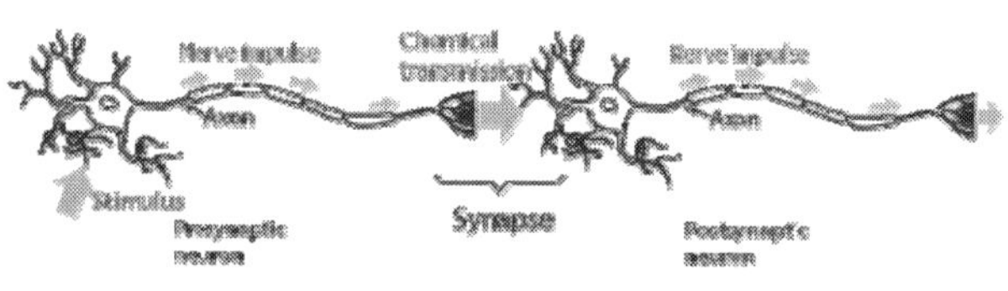

Figure 2. Chemical Transmission between synaptic gorges

nAChRs are highly sensitive to a class of biomolecules which contains chemical information, popularly termed as "Neurotransmitters" which is synthesized and released at the synaptic gorge mainly at the CNS. The latest finding gives the information that up to date there are several hundreds of neurotransmitters and neuropeptides have been identified (Ghijsen and Leenders 2005). All these neurotransmitters are responsible for chemical signaling. A single neuron has the potential to synthesize and release several neurotransmitters in a fraction of time frame (MacDermott *et al.* 1999).

The neurotransmitters are functions at different parts of the nervous systems and have different types of effects based on the type of chemical substances synthesized and targeted. For example, the neurotransmitter itself acts as a neuromodulator, in such a manner that some will be synthesized to initiate and promoted for the transmission of the chemical impulse, while others may focus on the inhibition mechanism of the same. Recently, the soluble Acetylcholine Binding Protein (AChBP) secreted by *Lymnaea stagnalis* at glial cells have been characterized as well (Brejc *et al.* 2001). In this case, the secretions of the protein complexes were modulated by neurotransmitters by themselves. The protein involved in functions, like in transport of neurotransmitter molecule to extra synaptic sites, allowing the interaction with, for instance, galial cells or other adjacent neurons and maintaining the concentration of the neurotransmitter at the synaptic gorge. Similar kind of neurotransmitters binding proteins were also exists at the Central Nervous System (CNS) in vertebrates (Kash *et al.* 2004; Farrant and Nusser 2005).

Studies on these ion channels reveal that nAChR were the target for several animal toxin substances. These substances were principally termed as neurotoxins, among which the most important toxin that targets to these ion channels were α-neurotoxin (Benie *et al.* 2000), a class of curare-mimetic neurotoxin which have the ability to paralyze the prey instantly. These peptide toxins were obtained from the wide variety of species from cone snails, spiders, scorpions, many-banded Taiwanese krait (*Bungarus multicintus*) snakes, Gila monster lizards and sea anemone possess the ability to act as promising leads and structural templates for novel therapeutic agents which spawned the field of pharmacology (Zingsheim, Barrantes *et al.* 1982). These bio-toxins targets to several skeletal muscles at neuromuscular junction particularly at presynaptic site. These neurotoxins binds to the target receptor molecule contains *phospholipase A_2* enzymes or these enzymes acts as an integral part of these neurotoxin, readily mediate the neurotoxic effects, results in the release of the neurotransmitter Acetylcholine (ACh). Other types of neurotoxins were also involved in this cholinergic neurotransmission which includes the neurotoxin fasciculin, from mamba (*Dendroaspis spp*) venom which inhibits the *acetylcholinestrase* activity at the neuromuscular junction as well as central synapse. The *κ*-neurotoxins from *Bungarus spp*, target to various types of neuronal subunits (e.g., $\alpha_2\beta_3$, $\alpha_4\beta_2$) (Zingsheim *et al.* 1982; Adams *et al.* 2003; Armishaw *et al.* 2006).

A class of α-neurotoxin from Elapid and Hydrophid snakes venom contains of about 60-74 residues which belongs to three-finger toxin superfamily on non-enzymatic polypeptides type known as α-Bungarotoxin (Harel *et al.* 2001). In general, the characteristics feature of all three-finger toxins and their distinctive structural conformation were arranged in three loops in the form of adjacent to each other. All these properties possess greater significance with respect to functional diversity and selectivity of molecular targets. Hence, despite the fingerprint of the similar fold, this three-finger toxin demonstrates a wide range of pharmacological activities. This includes both central and peripheral nervous neurotoxicity, cytotoxicity, cardiotoxicity, inhibition of enzymes such as *acetylcholinesterase* and *proteinases*, hyposensitive effects and platelet aggregation.

Another class of exclusive source of α-neurotoxins were also exists among the neurotoxin superfamily (Dutertre *et al.* 2004). These venoms are originated from many diverse species of marine cone snails, which represents a rich combinatorial like library of evolutionary selected neuropharmacologically active peptides called conotoxins. These conopeptides target towards a wide variety of ion channels, (e.g., Kv1.2 of VGIC superfamily and nAChR of LGIC superfamily). Particularly, snail toxins are too short when compared with snake toxins which is approximately of 12-30 residues in length and is highly rich in disulfide linkage in nature. One of the significant feature of this toxins are highly capable of sensing different types of ligand-binding interfaces of muscle nAChR as well as some that are selective for various subtypes of neuronal nAChRs.

Recent studies of the neuropsychopharmacological effects of ACh have focused primarily on nAChRs for their role in mediating neuromuscular and autonomic transmission. However, over the last decade, this trend has changed following preclinical and clinical studies indicating that neuronal nAChRs may have a substantial role in mediating antinociception, cognitive performance, modulating affect, and enhancing the release of other neurotransmitters (Jensen *et al.* 2005). Research related to nAChR by *insilico* approach such as Sequence analysis, Homology modeling, Molecular docking, Molecular dynamics, Computer Aided Drug Discovery, other broad area such as genomics, database, and studies on transcriptional factor is being carried out successfully (Sgrignani *et al.* 2009). However, three dimensional structure of nAChR is not available.

The crystal structure of α_7nAChR is not reported due to the presence of the transmembrane region which is coupled with the lipid bilayer. On the other hand, the crystal structure of Acetylcholine Binding Protein from *Lymnaea stagnalis* was solved by Brejc *etal* (2001) and the cryoelectron microscopic structure from Torpedo ray fish by Unwin (2005) acts as the structural template to model the α_7nAChR. Using this structure as the template, several theoretical model structures were constructed and investigated the active site on several other subunit of this receptor molecule. But still, the structure of α_7nAChR remains elusive.

In the Ligand Gated Ion Channel (LGIC) Database the nucleic and protein sequences of the subunits was available(Le Novere and Changeux 2001). Multiple sequence alignments can be generated, and phylogenetic studies of the super families are reported in this database. Finally, the atomic coordinates of subunits, or portion of subunits, were also provided. The LGIC Database redundancy is kept to a minimum, i.e. one entry per gene (Le Novere and Changeux 2001).

The nicotinic acetylcholine receptor is the best investigated Ligand-Gated Ion Channel (LGIC), and homology models of its ligand binding domain are not available. As an approach to investigate the function and subunit composition of nAChRs in native tissues, studies on structure-function relationships of α-conotoxins, small peptides from the venom of marine snails is carried over by Richard and Sebastien (2007) aimed at developing optimized selective peptide ligands as pharmacological tools (Nicke *et al.* 2004).

Epibatidine (EPB), an alkaloid isolated from the skin of the Ecuadorian poison frog, *Epipedobates tricolor* has attracted attention because of its exceptionally powerful analgesic properties and acts several hundred times greater than those of morphine, and nicotine. Although the substance is toxic, it does serve as a lead compound in the development of drugs for pain relief as well as treatment of disorders where pathogenesis involves nicotinic receptors. The work related to the isolation, effect on neuronal and neuromuscular nicotinic receptors, therapeutic potential, toxicity, nicotinic pharmacophore structural modifications related issues of epibatidine were also reported (Yogeeswari *et al.* 2006).

Reports on the structures of AChBP of *Lymnaea stagnalis* (Brejc *et al.* 2001) and on the theoretical models of heteropentameric subunits of nAChRs are available (Cheng *et al.* 2009). Those works were focused on investigating (i) the behavior of water molecule in the active site (ii) behavior of the protein molecule towards breathing motion (iii) demonstrating how the water molecule occupying the active site and used in the design of new ligands by comparing the positions of these sites with other recent structures (iv) conformational changes induced by the binding of ligand molecule in the active site (v) channel gating mechanism (vi) structural changes owing to ligand binding (vii) water density profiles. Further, several works related to the transmembrane domain of the channel to explore about the residue involved in the gating mechanism using lipid bilayer.

Review of literature revealed that the work on designing the rationalized lead molecule from agonist and competitive antagonist molecule is appears to be very meager. Thus present work focused α_7nAChR in response of neurotoxin and neurotransmitters in Structural Bioinformatics perspective.

Objectives

1. Homology modeling of Human Neuronal α_7nAChR.
2. Molecular interaction of agonist and competitive antagonist with Human Neuronal α_7nAChR.
3. *Insilico* Point mutations and Evolutionary Trace Analysis applied to Human Neuronal α_7nAChR.
4. Molecular Dynamics Studies of Human Neuronal α_7nAChR with Agonist and Antagonists.

Review of Literature

Ion channels are a distinct type of membrane transporter protein molecules, enables the transfer of inorganic ions through its central pore. These membrane proteins have been targeted for more than half of current drugs. These channels provide a unique opportunity to understand the physical basis of an integral membrane protein function at an atomic level (Sansom *et al.* 1998). The nicotinic acetylcholine receptor (nAChR) is the paradigm of Ligand-Gated Ion Channels

(LGIC) integral membrane proteins that mediate fast intracellular communications in response to neurotransmitters. The nAChR is the best characterized member of the LGIC superfamily, belonging to the Cys-loop superfamily that responds to the binding of neurotransmitter Acetylcholine (Cheng *et al.* 2007). nAChRs is the first ion channel and neurotransmitter membrane receptor and is one of the best known membrane protein which is involved in the signal transduction which was isolated and chemically identified (Salvaterra and Moore 1973).

History

nAChR is one of the significant ion channels involved in signal transmission between nerve cells and their targets at Central Nervous System (CNS) and Peripheral Nervous System (PNS) in vertebrates (Liu *et al.* 2008). The nicotinic receptors are widely distributed in pre-synaptic, post-synaptic or even axonic areas and they modulate the release of neurotransmitters by significant calcium influx in the presynaptic bouton (Itier and Bertrand 2001). nAChR holds a special place in the history of ion channels research; it was the first ion channels sequenced, purified, functionally reconstituted in synthetic lipid bilayers, cloned and recorded the electrical signal as a single open channel (Shen and Yakel 2009; Soriano *et al.* 2009; Tang *et al.* 2009). Furthermore, it is the only Ligand-gated Ion Channel (LGIC) to have an experimentally determined three-dimensional structure (Brejc *et al.* 2001; Unwin 2005). nAChR is physiological and pharmacologically significant ion channel and this three-dimensional structure used as a model for exploring structure-function relationship of LGIC superfamily (Barrantes 1997; Barrantes *et al.* 2000; Karlin 2002).

Classification & subunits

nAChRs are classified into muscarinic AChRs and nicotinic AChRs, which are named after the agonists derived from muscarine (*Amanita muscaria*) and nicotine (*Nicotiana tabacum*) respectively. There are 17 different nAChR subunits divided into two categories: muscle type α_1, β_1, δ, ε, γ and neuronal type (α_2- α_{10} and β_2-β_4). The nAChR channel is composed of five subunits, which can be subdivided into two group: subunits carrying the principle acetylcholine (ACh) binding site component (α_2-α_{10}) and subunit carrying the complementary component of the ACh binding site (non-α or β_2-β_4). The channels formed by these subunits can be either homomeric, consists of five subunits comprising the same type homomeric (α_7-α_9), or heterometic, where the neurotransmitter receptor consists of two or more different subunits. α_7nAChR are the only homomeric nicotinic receptors expressed in the human brain and is one of the two most abundantly expressed nicotinic receptor subtypes and the other type is heterodimer consisting of α_4 and β_2 subunits. Nicotinic receptors are always pentamers, with the subunits arranged symmetrically around a central receptor channel. The receptors always contain two or more alpha subunits, which are critical for acetylcholine binding (Itier and Bertrand 2001).

Function, dysfunction and diseases

A significant proportion of these membrane proteins are involved in diverse function like stabilizing synapse formation during development, learning, memory, neuronal survival and signal transduction particularly towards the nervous systems. The channel opening is induced by the neurotransmitters like Acetylcholine (ACh) (or Nicotine) binding. This results in the depolarization of the membrane, further leads to either modulation of the neuronal activity or muscle contraction. The various neurological diseases such as schizophrenia, Alzheimer's and Parkinson's diseases are believed to be caused due to the dysfunction of nAChR. In addition to the neurological diseases, these receptors play a major role in response to pain (Hogg and Bertrand 2007).

Physiological functions

The AChR family is implicated in several important physiological functions (Lloyd and Williams 2000). For instance, AChRs may directly or indirectly act on cognition, learning memory and attention, neurodegeneration, pain perception, reward anxiety and depression control, body temperature, protective response to stress (e.g., hypoxia) Cardiovascular and Gastrointestinal tract, as well as on muscle contraction and tone. From the pathological point of view, AChRs are involved in different neurological disorders including Alzheimer's and Parkinson's disease, schizophrenia, drug addiction, Tourette's syndrome, myasthenia gravis and myasthenia syndromes, depression, anxiety, ulcerative colitis, attention-deficit hyperactivity disorder, and neuroinflammation (Tuppo and Arias 2005) as well as on different types of epilepsies, including nocturnal lobe, juvenile myoclonic, and catamenial epilepsy (Lloyd and Williams 2000; Harel *et al.* 2001; Leonard and Bertrand 2001).

VARIOUS CONFORMATIONAL STATE OF LGIC

In particular, these biologically relevant properties were induced by the release and binding of specific neurotransmitters to its receptors. This binding takes several conformational changes in the receptor protein which takes several intermediate positions between the native and the open state. In general, three different conformational states were observed in these types of receptors. In broad-spectrum, many receptors prefer to be in resting state (R). The number of binding site of LGIC superfamily may vary, for example two for muscle type and five for homopentameric type of receptor in the closed form and still remains activated (A). All these change happens in the absence of the specific neurotransmitter and the receptor still remains activated (Jackson 1989). But in the presence of ligand or neurotransmitter the channel tends to open in rapid time frame from resting to activated state (R->A). In addition to activation of ion channel by neurotransmitters, the ion channels were activated by means of thermodynamics fluctuations to opening of ion channels but with much lower in probability. The prolonged binding of ligand to the ion channels leads to the desensitized state (D). The desensitized state has relatively higher affinity for the specific neurotransmitter as well as for other agonists and some antagonists than the resting state. Different receptors characteristics towards desensitization were found dissimilar (Edelstein *et al.* 1996). For instance the α_7nAChR subtypes reacts to the neurotransmitter and takes a faster desensitization position, but $\alpha_2\beta_2$ subtype practically does not desensitized at any stage of the presence of neurotransmitters. The way in which the receptor gets desensitized can be described in two different ways or pathways. In a ligand-bound complex, the receptor protein can reopen its loop region to get the ligand to wash out or the receptor return back to the resting state after the neurotransmitter dissociates from the pocket gradually. The desensitization processing is noted as a remarkable example for allosteric protein behavior. Thus, by physiologically the desensitization were considered to be major determinant at synaptic gorge.

CYS-LOOP OR NICOTINOID SUPERFAMILY

Among the members in LGIC superfamily, Cys-loop were highly conserved with a 13-residue spaced disulfide loop between 128-142 and 188-189 at the Extracellular (EC) domain of the α-subunit of nAChRs. This superfamily comprises four families of ion channels coupled receptors which are gated by specific neurotransmitters. This includes GABA type A and GABA type C receptors, Glycine receptors (GlyRs), $5HT_3$ receptors ($5HT_3$) receptors and both neuronal and muscle type nicotinic receptors (AChRs) [Fig. 3].

Apart from this conserved properties, some other structural and functional significant properties that appear to be common among the superfamilies of this type.

1. The sequence shares approximately 22-26% of homology among different subunits and 70% homology is obtained comparing with other subunits were observed (Le Novere *et al.* 1999). Thus the genetic evidence suggesting that all members evolved from the common ancestors.
2. The structural characteristics have been confirmed by X-ray crystallographic (Brejc *et al.* 2001) technique resolved at 2.7Å for EC domain derived from great pond snail *Lymnea stagnalis*.
3. The EC domain formed by ~206 residues which look like a beta propeller in architecture (Brejc *et al.* 2001). This domain predominantly preserves its secondary structure among their superfamily, by maintaining antiparallel β sheets which lies perpendicularly to the membrane surface. This model strongly acts as the structural template for EC portion of α_7 homomeric receptor by 22.4% homology.
4. The interface region which lies in between the subunits which acts as the active site of the nAChR. The binding studies of structures from nAChR with its agonists and competitive antagonists, it was confirmed that ligand binding sites are located at the interface region between the subunits (Schapira *et al.* 2002). The additional members in the superfamily like $GABA_A$, GlyRs also support this binding site location (Cheng *et al.* 2009).

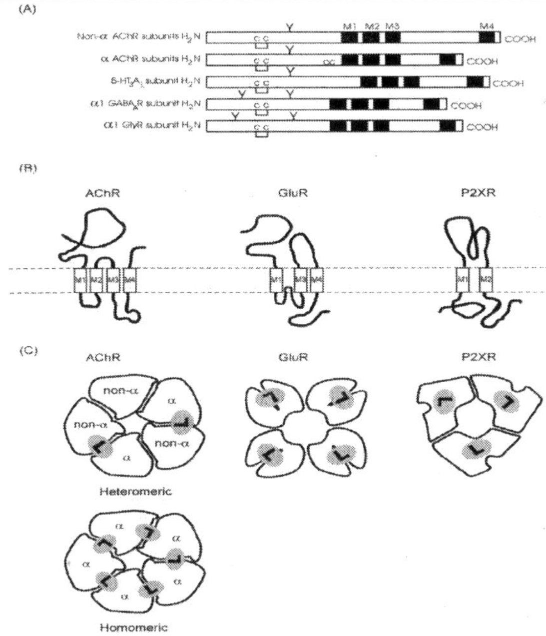

Figure 3: Schematic representation of the structures of members of Ligand-Gated Ion Channel. (A) Schematic illustration of the primary sequence of several subunits form members of the Ligand-Gated Ion Channel superfamily which includes the α type ($\alpha_2 - \alpha_9$) and non-α type (β_2- β_4, γ, ε and δ) subunits of the nAChR. (B) diagram of the tertiary organization of the AChR, the GluR, and the P2XR. The long N-terminal Extracellular Domain, the highly hydrophobic domain M1, M2, M3 and M4 and these Transmembrane are connected by a minor streaches, a Major Hydrophilic region facing the cytoplasm. (C) Schematic representation of the oligomeric organization of AChR, GluR and P2XR. The Hypotherical pentameric AChR is formed by two α subunits and three non- α chains. The two ligands binding sites (L) are located at the interfaces of one α subunit and one non-α chain. Regarding homomeric AChRs (eg. α_7, α_8, α_9) upto five binding sites may putatively exists.

5. The ligand binding site of this superfamily comprises many loop regions for efficient binding of agonists or antagonists. For this binding, the two subunits actively participate to make the binding complete and effective (Leonard and Bertrand 2001). The α subunit which donates

its residues for binding is known as principle component and the β subunit which donates for the same is known as complementary or secondary component domain.

6. Following this EC region, four TM segments (M1, M2, M3 and M4) arise for each subunit [Fig. 4 & 5]. Among the four TM helices M2 helix from each subunit which lies at the centre of this ion channel acts in the gating mechanism for the passage of the ions across the membrane. Rest of the helices (M1, M3 and M4) which lies outside M2 helices forming the helical bundle at the centre (Arias 1998; Arias 1998).
7. A "hydrophobic girdle" is formed at the middle of the M2 helix, formed by residues that are found to conserve throughout the superfamily. In particular this "hydrophobic girdle" residues involved in the gating mechanism (Unwin *et al.* 2002).
8. A dynamic mechanism called "ion channel gating", where agonist binding provokes a conformational change in the protein that finally leads the opening of the intrinsically-associated ion channel that is located for apart from the proper ligand binging domain. The main conclusion form these studies is that the chemical signal triggered by ACh binding is locally transmitted to the extracellular loop formed between M2 and M3 segments (Grosman *et al.* 2000; Grosman *et al.* 2000). The M2-M3 linker acts as a "conformational wave" that finally reaches the ion channel.
9. As discussed previously, the binding of ligand to the receptor takes numerous conformational states. Among which the desensitization state is the prolonged exposure of ligands to the receptors finally leads to refractory state where the ion channel will not open for agonist (Quick and Lester 2002).
10. A small cytoplasmic helix was found in between M3 and M4 of the TM helix (Cascio 2004). This varies in the length form 83-263. This region has the greatest sequence divergence among the superfamily members. This region is important for receptor modulation by phosphorylation and reverse phosphorylation mechanism.

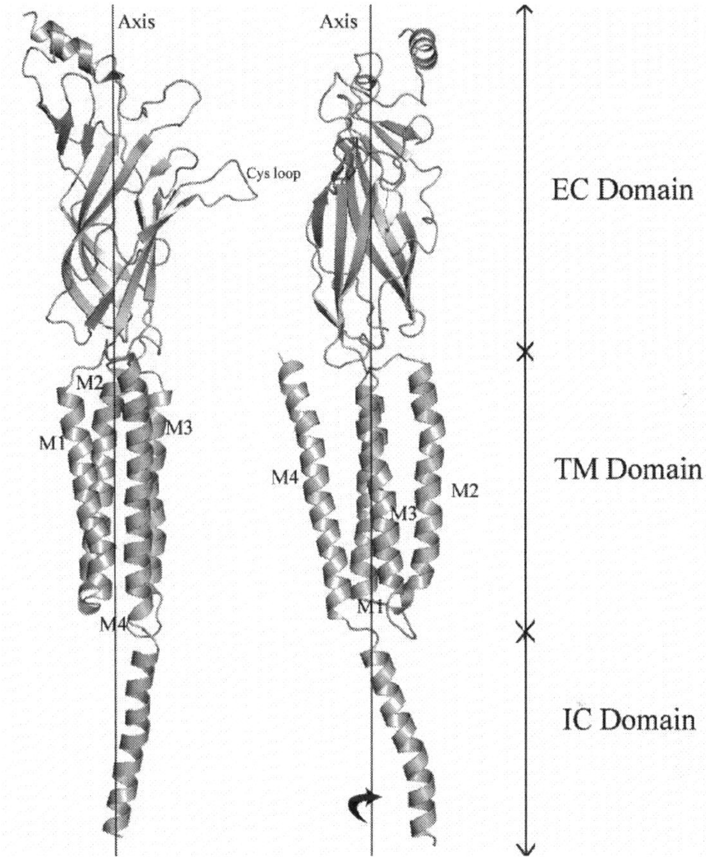

Figure 4: Ribbon diagram of a single subunit viewed parallel with membrane plane. The ECD is positioned at the top of the chain. The TM domain positioned at the centre of the chain. The intracellular domain positioned at the lower region of the chain. The four transmembrane helix bundles were displayed clearly, showing M2 helix facing inwards. From this it is understood that M2 forms principle domain in channel gating.

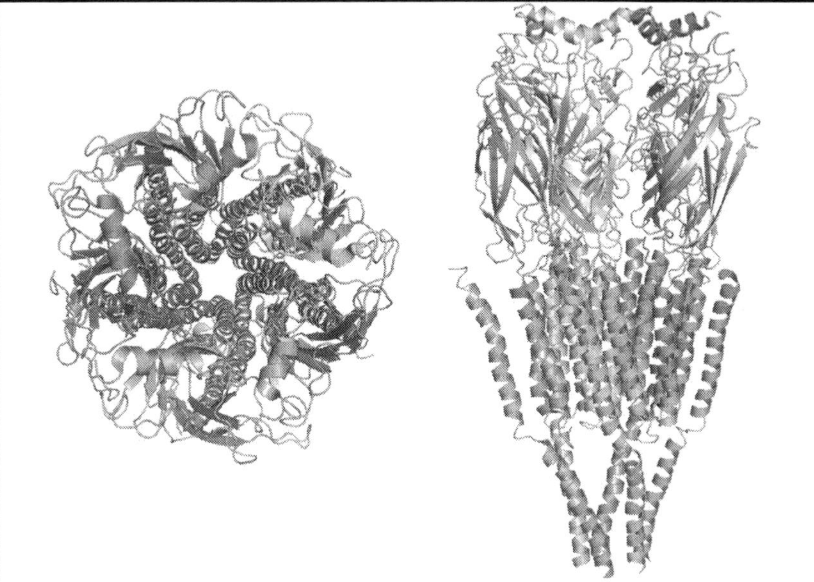

Figure 5: Ribbon diagrams of the whole nAChR receptor as viewed (a) from the synaptic cleft of top view and (b) parallel with the membrane plane on side view.

AChBP

The recent crystal structure of great pond snail (*Lymnaea stagnalis*) on Acetylcholine Binding Protein (AChBP) has showed a little success among LGIC superfamily. The subunit shares the sequence similarity of about ~22-27% with N-terminal Extracellular Domain (ECD) of nAChR and related channels, as well as having all the structural hallmarks that can be found in the α_7ECD. Thus AChBP can be used as a structural template for modeling the ECD of the nAChR and related channels. With this concordance, the structural similarity of AChBP can able to form a homopentamer, which is highly sensitive to the α-bungarotoxin (α-BTX) and other α_7 nAChR cholinergic ligands with comparable affinities, making it a suitable structural model for α_7-nAChR (Brejc *et al.* 2001).

Domains

nAChR subunit can be subdivided into two principal domains: the Extracellular (ECD) or Ligand Binding Domain (LBD) which carries the agonist and antagonist binding sites at the boundary between subunits and the transmembrane ion-pore domain that delineates a cation-specific axial channel with a central pore. Neuronal nAChR composed of combinations of nine α type (α_2 – α_{10}) and three non α type (β_2 – β_4) neuronal subunits rearranges to form a pentameric arrangement.

Types

nAChR exist in two type such as Muscle and Neuronal type. The muscle type nAChR exists with stoichiometric assembly $(\alpha_1)_2\beta_1\gamma\delta$ at neuromuscular junction. In the muscle nAChR, the ligand binding site is formed at the α/γ and α/δ interfaces, where the α subunit provides the principal binding surface (Dennis *et al.* 1988). This pentameric arrangement of this type nAChR appears to be the common drug target for muscle relaxants. The neuronal nAChR is an allosteric protein that exists as homomeric $(\alpha_7)_5$ or heteromeric assembly $(\alpha_4)_2(\beta_2)_3$ located at both pre and post synaptic nerve terminals. This acts as drug target for neurodegenerative diseases, nicotine addiction in smokers, effects of nicotine on cognition and memory (Dellisanti *et al.* 2007).

Active site

There are five nAChR ligand binding site, which are located at the five protomer interfaces (Karlin 2002). The ligand binding site is found in between the cleft region by a series of loops from the principle subunit (A) and a series of β-strands from the complementary subunit (B). The principle subunit of AB interface consists of residues comes from loop A (Tyr A89), loop B (Trp A143, A145) and loop C (Tyr A185, Cys187-188 and Tyr A192). The complementary part of this binding site is formed by β-strands from loop D (Trp B53, GlnB55), loop E (Arg B104, Val B106, Leu B112 and Met B114) and loop F (Tyr B164). Additional residues may also be involved in larger ligand binding such as toxins. The most likely access routes to the ligand-binding sites are from above or below the double-cysteine-containing loop C. This region buries the ligand binding site from the solvent, preventing access from the outside. In the case of accessing of larger ligand like d-tubocurarine, or toxins, it would require the binding site to be opened up by the C-loop region. But this requires a major structural rearrangement at the interface, which are less likely to occur (Brejc *et al.* 2001; Bourne *et al.* 2005; Janes 2005; Dellisanti *et al.* 2007).

Immunoglobulin architecture

Spectroscopic studies conducted on the recombinant amino-terminal Extracellular Domain (ECD) of various nAChR subunits which reveals that the ECD of nAChRs contains a high proportion of residues belonging to β-strands. The AChBP monomer has a short α-helix at the N-terminus, followed by two short 3_{10} helices and ten β-strands, termed β_1- β_{10}. The protein conforms to modified immunoglobulins (Ig) topology in which an inner β-sheet (composed of β_1, β_2, β_3 β_5, β_6 and β_8) is linked to an outer β-sheet (composed of β_4, β_7, β_9 and β_{10}) by means of a "Cys-loop" disulphide bridge and organize in a curled β-sandwich [Fig. 6]. The Cys-loop is a feature of the N-terminal ACh ion channel superfamily, and can be found between Cys 126 and Cys140 of α_7nAChR. The only contacts between subunits of a pentamer are the two dimer interfaces of each protomer (Bourne *et al.* 2005).

Glycosylation region

The residues forming the binding pockets are highly conserved between LGIC superfamily members, contradicting the low homology of the residues lining the interface between two protomers. In addition, the nAChR subunit contains three potential sites of N-linked glycosylation at N22, N68 and N111 within the ECD, although, due to their distance from the ligand binding sites, the absence of glycolsylation does not appear to affect ligand binding. The binding of either an agonist or antagonist to the binding pockets in the ECD may cause changes in the molecular structure of the receptor, which gets translated down to the TMD resulting in the opening or closing of the ion channel (Dellisanti *et al.* 2007).

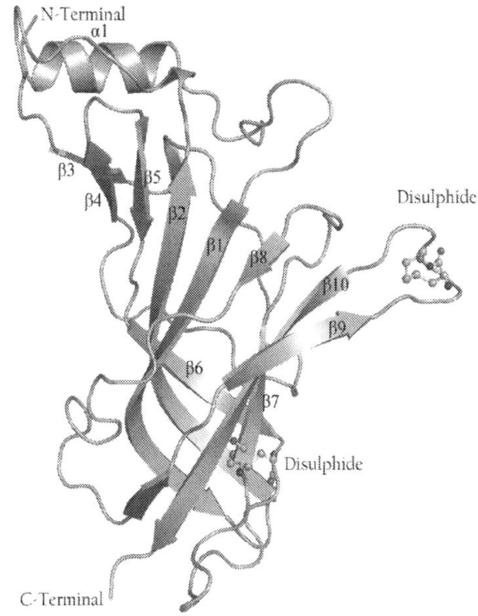

Figure 6: Theoretical structure of α_7nAChR protomer showing N-terminal and C-terminal. α_1 represents α helix. $\beta_{1\text{-}10}$ represents β strands. The disulphide bonds are displayed in ball and stick representation. In a complete structure, the N-terminal would point towards the synaptic gorge and C-terminal would enter the membrane at the bottom, continuing into the transmembrane domain.

TM and intracellular

The TMD of α_7nAChR is composed of four putative α-helices. Membrane Spanning Region (MSR) consisting of an average of 19-24 amino acids (MSR I-24, II-19, III-20 and IV-19). There exists a short cytoplasmic region between MSR I and II, and short extracellular region between MSR II and III. A large intracellular domain exists, however, between MSR III and IV (Unwin 2005).

Marine drugs

Several members from the AChR family are targets for the pharmacological action of different natural toxin (Arias 2000; Arias and Blanton 2000). The list of alkaloids that act as agonists includes (-) nicotine (obtained from the leaves of the tobacco plant *Nicotiana tabacum*), (+) anatoxin-a (obtained from the blue green algae Anabena flos-aquae), (-) Cystisine (obtained from the plant *Thermopsis alterniflora*), (+) epibatidine (obtained from the skin of the Ecuadorian frog *Epipedobates tricolor*), lobeline (obtained from the plant *Lobelia inflate*), and anabaseine (obtained from *Nemertine* marine worm species and form venom glands of certain ants). Among competitive antagonists we can name alkaloids such as d-tubocurarine (obtained from the bush *Chondrodendron tomentosum*), methyllcaconitine (obtained from different *Erythrina* plant species), snake polypeptides such as α- and κ-bungarotoxins [obtained from different Elapidae(e.g., the many – banded krait *Bunbarus multicintus*) and Hydrophiidae (sea snakes) species] and cobrotoxins (e.g., from *Naja naja siamensis*), as well as marine toxins such as lophotoxins (obtained from gorgonian corals such as *Lophogorgia* and *Pseudopterogorgia)*, neosurugatoxin (obtained from the Japanese ivory shell *Babylonia japonica*), as well as α- and αA- conotoxins (obtained from several *Conus species*). Finally, among non competitive Ψ-conotoxin PIIE (obtained from *C. purpurascens*). Although some toxins bind to different AChR in a nonspecific manner, several toxins present very high affinity and high specificity for certain receptor types, pointing out the importance for potential therapeutic uses.

Snake toxin

The peptide toxins from the species of cone snails, spiders, scorpions, snakes, Gila monster lizards and sea anemone possess the ability to act as promising leads and structural templates for novel therapeutic agents (Lewis and Garcia 2003). A snake toxin binds to the nAChR with high affinity and selectivity at postsynaptic nerve terminal. The first toxin which is used to characterize the nAChR is a long chain neurotoxin of which is the α-bungarotoxin (α-BTX) isolated from the banded krait snake (*Bungarus multicinctus*) venom (Dutertre and Lewis 2006). The long chain α-BTX with 74 amino acid residues and five disulfide bonds binds potently to both the muscle and neuronal α_7nAChR subtypes. We focus on α-Bungarotoxin, which targets nAChR as a competitive antagonist of acetylcholine and which inserts a finger at the interfaces. α-BTX exhibits high toxicity due to high affinity interaction with nAChR through its inhibition at the neuromuscular junction. The high affinity and specific interaction of α-BTX with nAChR has been considered to be of primary importance in the study of ligand binding sites of AChR, to investigate its strong competitive antagonistic activity (Harel *et al.* 2001).

Conotoxins

Another class of toxin, i.e., α-conotoxin [Fig. 7] is small disulphide-rich polypeotide components of the venoms of marine snails of the species *Conus*, and is specific inhibitors of nAChRs i.e., muscle nAChRs and/or specific subtypes of neuronal nAChRs in mammal (Armishaw *et al.* 2009). The α-conotoxin is antagonists of ACh Binding, and, being competitive inhibitors, they bind in the same region as ACh and prevent the channel from opening. In parallel with the two classes of nAChR, there are also two families of α-conotoxins, each favoring binding to one class over the other with a high degree of specificity (Armishaw and Alewood 2005).

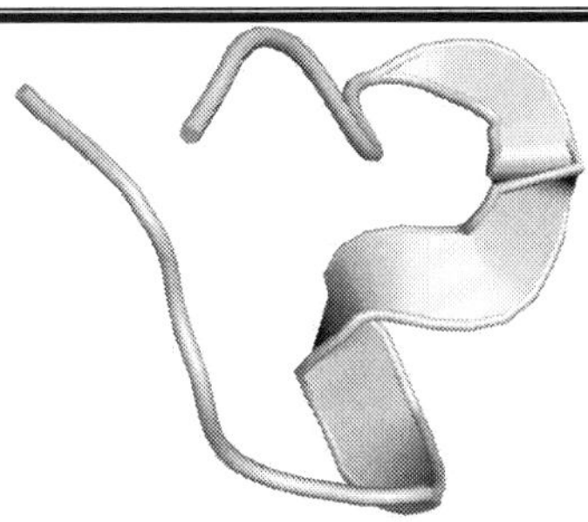

Figure 7: The Secondary structure representation of short α-neurotoxin, α-conotoxin.

Homology modeling

Based on the recent crystal structure from AChBP, the extracellular domain of $(\alpha_4)_2(\beta_2)_3$ and $(\alpha_1)_2\beta_1\gamma\delta$ were constructed using Homology Modeling approach by Le Novere *etal* revealed that the agonist binding site is globally conserved, and some specific positions should be crucial to pharmacological activity. The intersubunit chelating site for Ca^{2+} binding was also reported (Le Novere and Changeux 1995). In this study the distances between the binding residues were too large for a strong calcium site, where the typical distances between chelating atoms range form 3-5Å. However, the calcium site would reach its final conformation only in the open state, which could slightly differ from the putative desensitized state model (Smit *et al.* 2001).

Docking

The nicotinic receptors are known to react with chemically diverse compounds such as endogenous ligand acetylcholine, and naturally occurring compounds such as nicotine and alcohol (Prince and Sine 1999). The two neighbouring subunits and a disulphide bond between two adjacent cysteine residues contribute to the interaction of these compounds with receptors. The ligand binding site is highly characterized by aromatic and hydrophobic residues between the two adjacent subunits. These ligands are expected to bind at the same position at the interface region and tend to cause local conformational changes within the pentamer molecule (Celie *et al.* 2004).

The theoretical models of nAChR were also used to screen a large compound database and identify a new ligand candidate that could display subtype selectivity. Top scoring compounds were considered as good ligand candidates and were selected. In all these cases the predicted binding energies are better than nicotine or acetylcholine. The Van der Waals repulsions with $\alpha_4\beta_2$ and $\alpha_3\beta_2$ nAChRs remain small, and within the accuracy limit of Van der Waals energy prediction were reported (Holladay *et al.* 1997).

For the treatment of diseases involving nAChRs, drugs must be designed with a high level of selectivity towards only one of these classes or subclasses (in cases of neuronal receptors) (Janes 2003). The study relating to neuromuscular and neuronal specific α-conotoxin, SI and EpI are important. A significant difference can be seen in the shapes of these molecules, which reflect topological features of the different types of target receptor subunit. When compared the backbone conformation, there was clearly a considerable difference observed in over all shape between C-terminal regions of the molecules. This difference is a reflection of the larger number of residues in the neuronal versus the neuromuscular conotoxin between the third and fourth cysteine residues. This study suggests that the neuronal ACh binding site might be longer and narrower than its neuromuscular counterpart (Janes 2005).

Molecular dynamics

Molecular dynamics simulations of biological membranes in pure lipid bilayers are extending the understanding of both optimal simulations procedures and the detailed structural dynamics of lipids in these systems. Simulation methods established using simple bilayer-embedded peptides are being extended to a wide range of membrane transports, membrane proteins and membrane protein models, and are beginning to reveal some of the complexities of membrane protein structural dynamics and their relationship to biological function (Forrest and Sansom 2000).

Membrane transport constitutes one of the most fundamental processes in all living cells with proteins as major players. Proteins as channels provide highly selective diffusive pathways gated by environmental factors, and as transporters furnish directed, energetically uphill transport consuming energy. X-ray crystallography of channels and transporters furnishes a rapidly growing number of atomic resolution structures, permitting molecular dynamics (MD) (Khalili-Araghi *et al.* 2009).

MD provides a useful way to examine the dynamic behavior of proteins and indeed has been recently applied to model of α_7nAChR (Kandt *et al.* 2007), where focus was on examining the large-scale motion of the protein thought to be related to gating in nAChRs. Studies focused largely on the dynamics of the residues and water in the binding pocket of the nAChR great in detail (Kandt *et al.* 2005). The details of interaction in a complex between antagonists such as long chain α-neurotoxin and α-conotoxin with nicotinic acetylcholine receptor (nAChR) and conformational changes induced by these antagonists were also reported. Upon binding of α-neurotoxin, ligand bounded nAChR is less dynamic in certain domains than the apo form of the conotoxin-nAChR complex. A critical interaction in the binding site such as the salt bridge formation between K145-D200 in the neurotoxin-nAChR complex is further stabilized during the MD simulations (Nasiripourdori *et al.* 2009).

Studies pointing to nAChR on Brownian dynamics simulations of Na^+ permeation through the open channel demonstrated a current-voltage relationship that was consistent with experimental data on the conducting state of $\alpha_4\beta_2$ nAChR. Besides establishment of the well-equilibrated closed- and open-channel $\alpha_4\beta_2$ structural models, the MD simulations on these models provided valuable insights into critical factors that potentially modulate channel gating. Rotation and tilting of TM2 helices led to changes in orientations of pore-lining residue side chains. Without concerted movement, the reorientation of one or two hydrophobic side chains could be enough for channel opening. The closed- and open-channel structures exhibited distinct patterns of electrostatic interactions at the interface of extracellular and transmembrane domains that might regulate the signal propagation of agonist binding to channel opening (Haddadian *et al.* 2008).

Modeling and simulation studies of M2 helices have also been performed. Law *etal* (Law *et al.* 2000) performed MD simulations on the pore-lining M2 helix of the nAChR to explore how its structure and dynamics changed as a function of environment. In water, the M2 helix partially unfolds to form a molecular hinge in the vicinity of a central Leu residue that has been implicated in the mechanism of ion-channel gating (Revah *et al.* 1991; Nowak *et al.* 1995). In a phospholipid bilayer, either as a single transmembrane helix or as part of a pentameric helix bundle, the M2 helix shows less flexibility, but still exhibited a kink in the vicinity of the central Leu. The single M2 helix tilted relative to the bilayer normal by 12°, in agreement with solid state NMR data (Opella *et al.* 1999).

Later Law *etal* (Sansom *et al.* 2002) have performed an extended (>15ns) MD simulation of a pentameric bundle (M2δ5) model of the pore-lining region of the nAChR in a POPC bilayer to explore the conformational dynamics of the channel assembly. On the time scale of the simulation, the bundle remains stable, with the polar pore-ling side-chains remaining exposed to the lumen of the channel. Fluctuations at the helix termini, and in the helix curvature, result in closing/opening transitions at both mouths of the channel, on a time scale of ~10ns. Recent NMR and modeling studies of the M2 helix bundle from the GlyR (Tang *et al.* 2002) have also suggested that changes in M2 helix packing may correlate with channel opening and closing.

Materials and Methods:

Sequence Alignment:

The protein sequence of LBD of Human neuronal α_7nAChR was retrieved from the UniProtKB/Swiss-prot (P36544) (Apweiler *et al.* 1997; Bairoch and Apweiler 1997; Bairoch and Apweiler 1997) database release 54.2. The sequence obtained from Swiss-prot was subjected to NCBI-BLAST (Altschul *et al.* 1990; Altschul and Lipman 1990) and to PSIPRED, a Protein Structure Prediction Server (McGuffin *et al.* 2000; McGuffin and Jones 2003) to extract information about suitable structural templates as well as secondary structure elements. The protein sequence of LBD-α_7nAChR and AChBP (P58154) was aligned using EBI-Align server (Lombard *et al.* 2002; Stoesser *et al.* 2002).

Homology Modeling of LBD-α_7nAChR:

The Modeller9v2 software (Sali and Blundell 1993) was employed in the construction of three-dimensional theoretical model for LBD of α_7nAChR for all five subunits. These five subunits were assembled to form a homopentamer. The final pentamer was generated using InsightII (Accelrys, San Diego, USA) on Silicon Graphics Workstation based on the initial equivalencies information from EBI-DaliLite (Holm and Park 2000). The theoretical model of pentamer was subjected to SYBYL 7.1 (Tripos Inc., St. Louis, MO, USA) package for correcting the bumps and stereochemistry at the interface regions. The energy minimization calculations were performed using SYBYL with 100 iterations which did not significantly alter the initial model. The geometric inaccuracies of the theoretical model were evaluated by subjecting the model to RCSB ADIT Validation server, an online web interface which provides validation reports from PROCHECK (Morris *et al.* 1992; Laskowski *et al.* 1993). Furthermore, the theoretical model (α_7nAChR) of this pentamer was structurally aligned with the experimental structure (AChBP) and rendered using PyMOL [].

Docking of competitive antagonist with theoretical structure α_7nAChR:

The structure of snake toxin α-Bungarotoxin (PDB code: 1HC9) which is a competitive antagonist of LBD-α_7nAChR was obtained from Protein Data Bank (Berman *et al.* 2000; Berman *et al.* 2000). The toxin was docked to the interface region of the theoretical structure of LBD-α_7nAChR using the docking program 3D-Dock (Katchalski-Katzir *et al.* 1992; Gabb *et al.* 1997). The total Accessible Surface Area (ASA) was calculated for bound and unbound coordinates by online web interface VADAR (Willard *et al.* 2003). The buried surface and inter-subunit possible hydrogen bonding network of the complexes were determined by subjecting the bound complexes to the online web interface WHATIF (Vriend 1990) provided by CMBI. The bound complexes were subjected to Protein-Protein Interaction Server (v1.5) (Jones and Thornton 1995) to analyze the protein interface of complexes.

Docking of small agonist with theoretical structure α_7nAChR:

The ligands such as acetylcholine and nicotine were obtained from PubChem database. These ligands were docked to the binding site of the theoretical model of pentamer with widely used program AutoDock3 (Goodsell *et al.* 1996; Morris *et al.* 1996; Osterberg *et al.* 2002; Morris *et al.* 2008). The interaction between the ligands and pentamer were analyzed using Ligplot (Wallace *et al.* 1995) and LPC-CSU server (Sobolev *et al.* 1999).

Retrieving Small molecules and processed for interaction with theoretical structure **α_7nAChR**

The Agonists and Antagonists [Table 1] were retrieved from PubChem database. These small molecules were retrieved in standard 2D SDF format. These molecules were converted into 3D by applying MMCF force field and subsequently minimized up to 50 iterations using VLifeMDS suite [VlifeSciences, Pune].

Molecular docking of agonist and antagonist with theoretical structure α_7nAChR

The processed agonist and the antagonist molecules were subjected to docking with the theoretical structure of α_7nAChR using widely used docking program AUTODOCK4 (Morris *et al.* 2009). The docking was performed for all the small molecules by keeping the ligands as flexible. The grid was placed at the interface region of the theoretical model of α_7nAChR.

Polar hydrogen was added by using the Hydrogen module in AutoDock Tools (ADT) for α_7nAChR dimer; followed by assigning Kollman united atom partial charges. The docking of α_7nAChR with the agonist and antagonist was carried out using the empirical free energy function and the Lamarckian genetic algorithm, applying a standard protocol with an initial population of 150 randomly placed individuals. A maximum number of 2.5×10^7 energy evaluations, a mutation rate of 0.02, and a cross over rate of 0.08, where the average of the worst energy was calculated over a window of the previous 10 generations, were involved to standardize the protocol. Genetic Algorithm of 100 independent docking cycles was carried out for each ligand. The grid maps representing the proteins in the actual docking process were calculated with AutoGrid. The grids were chosen to be sufficiently large to include the active site. The dimensions of the grids were thus 60Å x 60Å x 60Å, with a spacing of 0.536Å between the grid points. Results were clustered according to the 1.0 Å Root-Mean Square Deviations (RMSD) criterions. The entire small molecule bound to α_7nAChR was examined for binding energy and also for specific and non-specific interacting residues. The non-specific residues which appear to be common for all the docking was considered as class-specific residues. The molecules with lesser binding energy were ignored for further analysis.

Those residues were mapped on the sequence alignment and mutated on the theoretical model of α_7nAChR. The ligands were once again docked using AUTODOCK with α_7nAChR by keeping the ligand non-rotatable (freeze) by reducing the torsion angle to zero. The same protocol was followed for the following consecutive dockings.

Insilico Point Mutation

The theoretical model is subjected to three different types of mutation, based on the property of the residues. These three different mutated models were subjected to energy minimization to reduce the geometrical inaccuracies occurred due to mutation.

These mutated models were again docked using AUTODOCK by keeping the ligands non-rotatable. All the three different mutated theoretical models complexed with ligands were examined for the interaction of the mutated (non-specific residues) residues with the ligands. The ligand bound complexes were analyzed for bonded (H-bond) and non-bonded interaction using the in-house program Interactor and AUTODOCK for non-specific residues for all the three types of mutated complex and is compared with the wild type complexes.

Table 1: List of Agonists and Antagonists molecules used for docking with α_7nAChR. The structures were retrieved from PubChem database.

S.No	CID	Agonists
1	187	Acetylcholine
2	942	Nicotine
3	204966	Bromoacetylcholine
4	2551	Carbamylcholine
5	8425	Codeine
6	854023	Epibatidine
7	22407	Cyticine
8	9651	Galanthamine
9	8765	Physostigmine
S.No	**CID**	**Antagonists**
10	3604	Hexamethonium
11	9714	Mecamylamine
12	586269	4-(N-Maleimido)benzyltrimethylammonium
13	586270	4-(N-Maleimido)phenyltrimethylammonium
14	9778	Phencyclidine
15	222907	Dihydro-beta-erythroidine
16	108179	Lophotoxin
17	6000	d-Tubocurarine

Evolutionary Trace Analysis

The homologous protein sequences of nicotinic nAChRs [Table 2] were retrieved from UniProtKB/Swiss-Prot (Apweiler *et al.* 1997; Bairoch and Apweiler 1997; Bairoch and Apweiler 1997) respectively. All these homologous sequences were subjected to Evolutionary Trace analysis which was performed using TraceSuiteII server (Innis *et al.* 2000).

This eventually distributes the sequences into ten different partitions over the phylogenetic tree ranging from P01-P10 inorder to increase the Evolutionary Trace Cutoff (ETC) value by using the *TraceGroups*. For each partition, a trace procedure was completed automatically by these following steps respectively. (I) the protein sequences was connected by a common node with evolutionary time greater than the given ETC were clustered together; (II) A consensus sequences was generated for each group to distinguish between conserved and non-conserved positions; (III) A trace was generated by comparing the aligned consensus sequences for all the clusters associated with a given partition; thus, residues were classified into three types: Conserved, Class-specific and Neutral.

Residues that are important to function, but contribute more to the functional specificity of a particular subgroup of proteins in the family are likely to be conserved, but not invariant. Therefore, even though they might undergo mutations, the rate of mutations is still minimal. The class-specific residue denotes residues occupying a strictly conserved, located in the sequences alignment, but differing in the nature of their conservation between various subgroups. This information obtained by the ET method can be then mapped on to the known protein structures, thus allowing us to identify clusters of important amino acids and to distinguish between buried and exposed residues.

By comparing the consensus sequences a 'trace' is generated briefly for group of proteins that originate from a common node in a phylogenetic tree and are characterized by a common Evolutionary Time Cut-off (ETC).

Table 2: Homologues sequences of α_2, α_3, α_4, α_7 and α_9 of neuronal nAChRs were retrieved form SwissProt for Evolutionary Trace Analysis.

S.No	α_2		α_3		α_4		α_7		α_9	
	Source	**Swissprot Id**	**Source**	**Swissprot Id**	**Source**	**Swissprot Id**	**Source**	**Swissprot Id**	**Source**	**Swissprot Id**
1	HUMAN	Q15822	HUMAN	P32297	HUMAN	P43681	HUMAN	P36544	HUMAN	Q9UGM1
2	RAT	P12389	RAT	P04757	RAT	P09483	RAT	Q05941	RAT	P43144
3	MOUSE	Q91X60	MOUSE	Q8R4G9	MOUSE	O70174	MOUSE	P49582		
4	CHICK	P09480	CHICK	P09481	CHICK	P09482	CHICK	P22770	CHICK	Q9PTS8
5	PANTR	Q5IS52	BOVIN	Q07263	PANTR	Q5IS77	BOVIN	P54131		
6			CARAU	P18845	MUSPF	Q19AE6	MACMU	Q866A2		

Molecular Dynamics

Based on the clusters generated and the binding energy from the docking studies, one ligand bound protein complex was selected from each agonist and antagonists for Molecular Dynamics simulation. Galanthamine was selected for agonists group and Lophotoxin was selected form antagonists group respectively.

MD simulation was carried out with GROMACS v 3.1.2 (Van Der Spoel *et al.* 2005; Kutzner *et al.* 2007) suite of programs using the Gromacs force field [33] using NPT and periodic boundary conditions by four steps. The MD simulations were run on a 124 CPU quadrome cluster.

1. Protein Preparation

The topologies were generated for both Galanthamine and Lophotoxin using PRODRG server (Schuttelkopf and van Aalten 2004). Each of the complexes was placed in the centre of a 41 Å x 41 Å x 41 Å cubic box of approximately at 0.9 Å with Simple Point Charge (SPC/E) water molecules. Six NA^+ counterions were added to replace the solvent bulk of the protein-ligand/water complexes to maintain the electro neutrality of the system.

2. Energy Minimization

Each system was energy-minimized until convergence using steepest descents algorithm. During minimization, the Berendsen [35] temperature coupling and Berendsen pressure coupling (the coupling constants were both set to 0.1) were used to keep the system in a stable environment (300K). The minimization was carried out for about 1000 iterations to reduce the large force generated due to added hydrogen and broken hydrogen bond network, and also to reduce structure distortion of the system. The system was converged in 600 steps. This results in a structure that is stable enough for running a full simulation later.

3. Position Restraint

An equilibrium run was performed for about 20ps to avoid unnecessary distortion of the protein, where all the heavy protein atoms are restrained to their starting positions, while the solvent water is applied to relax around the structure. Remaining parameters were identical to energy minimization steps. The temperature and pressure were controlled with the Berendsen weak coupling algorithm.

4. Production Run

The Molecular Dynamics simulations of dimeric α_7nAChR with and without ligands were carried out for 2 and 10 ns each. During the production run Parinello-Rahman [36] algorithm was used for pressure coupling and temperature was coupled at 300K. The long range Electrostatics was calculated with the Particle Mesh Ewald (PME) [38, 39] method with the cutoff 6. The LINear Constraint Solver algorithm [40] was used to constrain bond lengths.

5. Analyzing the trajectory

The MD trajectories were analyzed using several inbuilt analyzing options from GROMACS.

a. Analyzing RMSF

The root mean square fluctuation (RMSF) for each residue in the modeled structure was calculated for the 10ns run each. RMSF gives a measure of the relative standard fluctuations for each residue in α_7nAChR. It is calculated by fitting to a reference structure, in this case from the structure at 0ns to that provided by the 10ns trajectory.

b. Analyzing Radius of gyration.

The Radius of gyration about the channel axis (R_g) is defined as

$$R_g = [\ \sum_i m_i r_i^2 / \sum_i m_i\ ]^{1/2}$$

where m_i is the mass of Cα atom i, $r_i = (X_i^2 + Y_i^2)^{1/2}$ is the distance of atom i from the central axis of the channel (the z axis), and the sum is over all Cα atoms in the protein.

c. Analyzing protein-ligand interactions

Protein-ligand interactions at active site region of the protein were measured using the presence of hydrogen bonds and the neighboring residues. Existing and new hydrogen bonds formed between the segments were recognized by a pure distance filter. If two nucleophiles (nitrogen and oxygen atoms) were within 3.2Å to each other, a potential hydrogen bond was recorded. Nucleophiles, in the backbone and side chain (C, O, N, OD1, OD2, OE1, OE2, NE1 and NE2) were considered for the distance calculations between the regions of interest using an in-house program called INTERACTOR (R.Sowdhamini, unpublished results). No distinction was made between weak and strong hydrogen bonds or whether they connect backbone or side chain atoms. Interesting regions are defined elsewhere. In addition to that Protein-ligand interactions were visualized with LigPlot (Wallace *et al.* 1995) and Pymol [42].

d. Analyzing water mediated interactions

Further, water mediated interactions that are mediated by neighboring water molecules, captured during the simulation, and was also monitored. No specific consideration was made to include only conserved waters. The primary shell of waters was recognized using an in-house program called STRIPWATER (R.Sowdhamini, unpublished results). These waters were identified by the condition that the oxygen atom should be within hydrogen bonding distance (≤3.2A) of at least one protein nucleophile within any of the three regions of interest.

Result and Discussion

4.1. Homology modeling of Human Neuronal α_7nAChR.

Sequence alignment of nAChR and AChBP protomer:

The full length protein sequence of α_7nAChR (502 residues) was extracted from SwissProt database, out of which N-terminal of α_7nAChR accounts for about 208 residues [Table 3]. The main reason behind this selection was LBD acts as the crucial region of agonist and competitive antagonist binding site at the interface region, which is highly conserved among their superfamilies [Fig.8].

```
                          α1                                β1
1I9B        -------FDRADILYNIRQTSRPDVIPTQRDRPVAVSVSLKFINILEVNE 43
α7nAChR     -------FQRKLYKELVKNYNPLERPVANDSQPLTVYFSLSLLQIMDVDE 43
                   **:*     ::: .  :    :: .:*::* .**.:::*::*:*

                 β2         η1             β3  η2      β4
1I9B        ITNEVDVVFWQQTTWSDRTLAWNSSHSP--DQVSVPISSLWVPDLAAYN- 90
α7nAChR     KNQVLTTNIWLQMSWTDHYLQWNVSEYPGVKTVRFPDGQIWKPDILLYNS 93
             .: : . :* * :*:*: * ** *. *   . * .* ..:* **:   **

               β5    β5'     β6     β6'                β7
1I9B        AISKPEVLTPQLARVVSDGEVLYMPSIRQRFSCDVSGVDTESG-ATCRIK 139
α7nAChR     ADERFDATFHTNVLVNSSGHCQYLPPGIFKSSCYIDVRWFPFDVQHCKLK 143
            * .: :.      . * *.*.  *:*.    : ** :.     . .   *::*

                   β8                         β9
1I9B        IGSWTHHSREISVDPTTENSDDSEYFSQYSRFEILDVTQKKNSVTYSCCP 189
α7nAChR     FGSWSYGG--WSLDLQMQEADISGYIPN-GEWDLVGIPGKRSERFYECCK 190
            :***::  .    *:*    :::* * *:.: ..::::::. *:..   *.**

                β10
1I9B        EAYEDVEVSLNFRKKG 205
α7nAChR     EPYPDVTFTVTMRRRT 206
            *.* ** .::.:*::

                 1I9B        - Lymnaea stagnalis
                 α7nAChR     - Homo sapiens
```

Figure 8: Sequence alignment of human α_7nAChR with AChBP of *Lymnea stagnalis*. α_1 represents α helix. β_{1-10} represents β strands. η_{1-2} represents 3_{10} Helix. Residues highlighted in box represents binding site residues. The alignment generated using EBI-Align which shows 22.4% sequence identity.

Table 3: Sequence information for LBD of nAChR length 208 residues was selected form *Homo sapiens*. AChBP from *Lymnaea stagnalis* length 205 residues acts as the structural template for nAChR.

Protein	SwissProt ID	Sequence length	Source	PDB code
nAChR (Target)	P36544	208	*Homo sapiens*	
AChBP (Template)	P58154	205	*Lymnaea stagnalis*	1I9B

The PSIPRED as well as NCBI-BLAST results suggested the Acetylcholine Binding Protein (PDB code: 1I9B) (Brejc *et al.* 2001) of snail refined at 2.7Å resolutions as a structural template and which has 22.4% sequence identity with α_7nAChR. Moreover, there was good agreement between the secondary structural elements of both sequences in the crucial regions (Russell *et al.* 1997).

The monomeric sequence of nAChR and AChBP were aligned using the EBI-Align server. On the basis of several secondary structure prediction tools, it is suggested that the N-terminal region of α_7nAChR mostly comprises series of β strands exhibiting an immunoglobulin fold topology (Corringer *et al.* 2000).

Model of human α_7 Pentamer:

Based on the alignment generated by EBI-Align, the program MODELLER9v2 was used to construct the theoretical structure of LBD of α_7nAChR using the crystal structure of the AChBP monomer as the template. This approach is still the best available when a homolog of the target is known (Orengo *et al.* 1999). Modeling of one subunit generated 20 different models, out of which a structure with minimum energy value was, selected [Fig. 9]. The model composed of an N-Terminal α-helix followed by ten strands that form a β-sandwich and comprise an immunoglobulin fold. A di-sulphide bond is formed between CYS126–CYS140. As expected the model of ECD of the human α_7nAChR does not exhibit major differences with the template. Although several parts of the sequence of the α_7nAChR ECD shows lower homology with the template the 13 residue Cys-loop is highly conserved among the superfamily, adopts similar structure to that of the template.

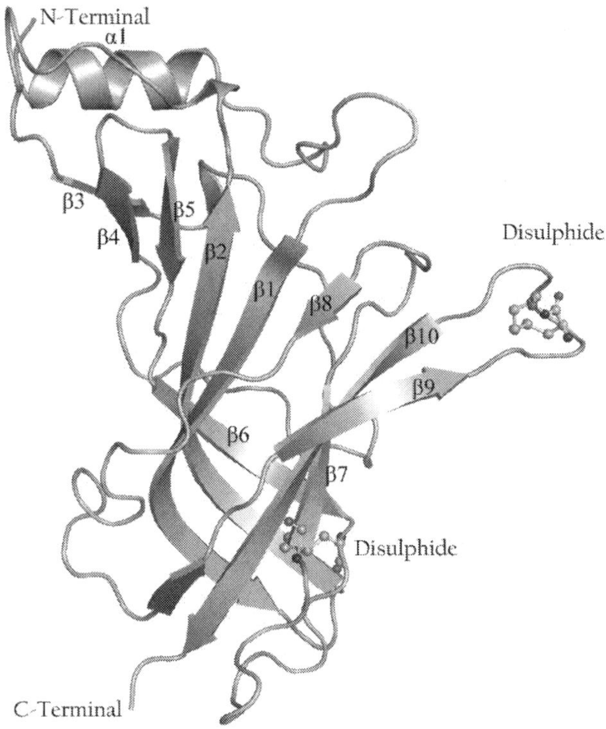

Figure 9: Theoretical structure of α_7nAChR protomer showing N-terminal and C-terminal. α_1 represents α helix. $\beta_{1\text{-}10}$ represents β strands. The disulphide bonds are displayed in ball and stick representation. In a complete structure, the N-terminal would point towards the synaptic gorge and C-terminal would enter the membrane at the bottom, continuing into the transmembrane domain.

The EBI-DaliLite server was used to obtain the structural superimposition of the residues of the experimentally available monomer and theoretically obtained structure. Based on the information provided by EBI-DaliLite, 5 fold symmetry of the theoretical structure of nAChR was generated using InsightII [Fig. 10] using the pentameric crystal structure as the reference structure. The resulting structure is the entire pentameric theoretical structure of LBD of α_7nAChR. On the other hand the structure is fully packed with steric clashes and geometric inaccuracies with higher energy which is supposed to be highly unstable, which is unsuitable for further exploration of the theoretical channel α_7nAChR.

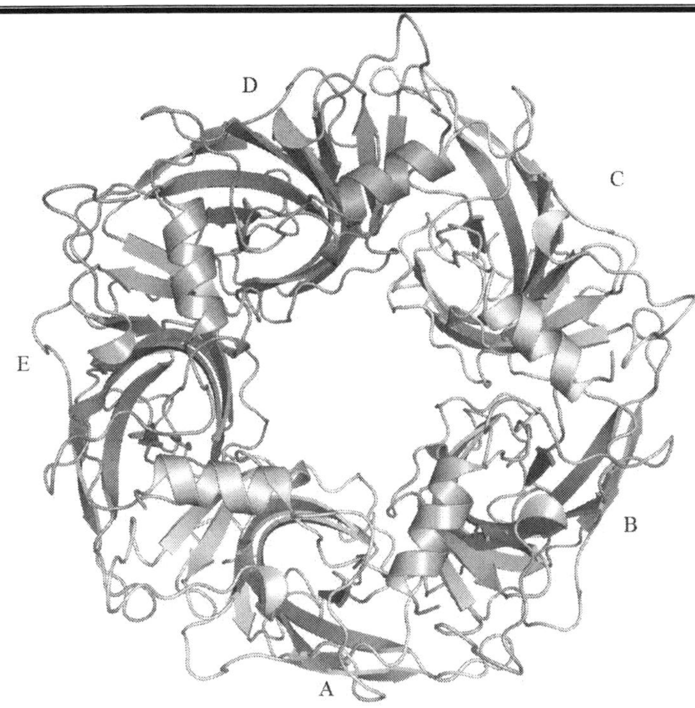

Figure 10: Secondary structure representation of α_7nAChR pentamer viewed down the fivefold axis. Each of the five identical subunits is rendered in a different color and labeled A, B, C, D, and E. A ligand binding site is formed at each interface, with A forming the (+) side and B forming the (-) side, and so on for B-C, C-D, D-E, E-A.

Subsequently, the energy minimization was carried out by using SYBYL 7.1 software using Tripos Force field. The pentamer was subjected to 100 iterations that remove the steric clashes at the subunit interfaces. This brings the pentameric structure with global minimum with the total clearance of the steric clashes.

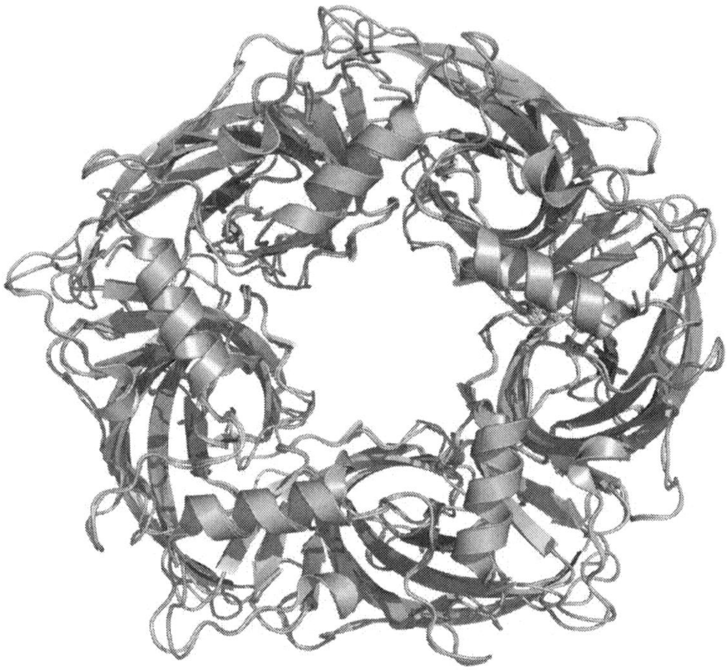

Figure 11: Superimposition of pentameric α_7nAChR (light green) and pentameric AChBP (orange) constructed using PyMol. Secondary structure conservation with theoretical model nAChR (light green) on AChBP (orange) is shown. Root Mean Square Deviation was observed to be 0.87Å.

The streochemical quality was examined using Procheck, probably the most powerful determinant of the quality of the protein coordinates. The quality of the Ramachandran plot was reasonably good when compared to that of the template structure which supports the reliability of the theoretical model. The average pairwise RMS fit of the Cα coordinates of these theoretical and experimental structures was 0.873 Å [Fig. 11] indicating a strong structural conservation seen among them and similarly in the structural folds.

The major segment of the α_7nAChR sequence involved in the binding site was in good consensus with the template AChBP, while the part of the sequence located away from the binding pocket showed less conservation with the template. Hence, the superimposition results indicated that, the Structurally Conserved Regions (SCRs) and the Structural Variable Region (SVRs) are quite similar with respect to the target (α_7nAChR) and the template (AChBP). The key residues of AChBP and the theoretical model of α_7nAChR in the interface region were observed to be conserved [Table 4].

Table 4: Interface residues

S.No	AChBP	nAChR
1	A-TYR89	A-TYR91
2	A-TRP143	A-TRP147
3	A-HIS145	A-TYR149
4	A-TYR185	A-TYR186
5	A-CYS187	A-CYS188
6	A-CYS188	A-CYS189
7	A-TYR192	A-TYR193
8	B-TRP53	B-TRP53
9	B-GLN55	B-GLU55
10	B-ARG104	B-LEU107
11	B-VAL106	B-ASN109
12	B-LEU112	B-GLN115
13	B-MET114	B-LEU117
14	B-TYR164	B-TYR166

Residues present at the corresponding interface region of AChBP and theoretical model of nAChR.

Ligand Binding Domain interface:

In the case of model of human α_7nAChR, the pentameric nAChR subunits were arranged with the presence of clefts at the interface region. This cleft lines up with residues which are involved in ligand binding. The cleft found in ligand binding domain was assembled by a series of loops from the principal face (+ side) of one subunit and a series of β-strands from the complementary face (- side) of the adjacent subunit. The principle side chain residues are involved from loop A

(TYR 91), loop B (TRP 147, TYR 149), loop C (TYR 186, CYS 188, CYS 189, TYR 193) and the complementary side chain residues from loop D (TRP 53, GLU 55), loop E (LEU 107, ASN

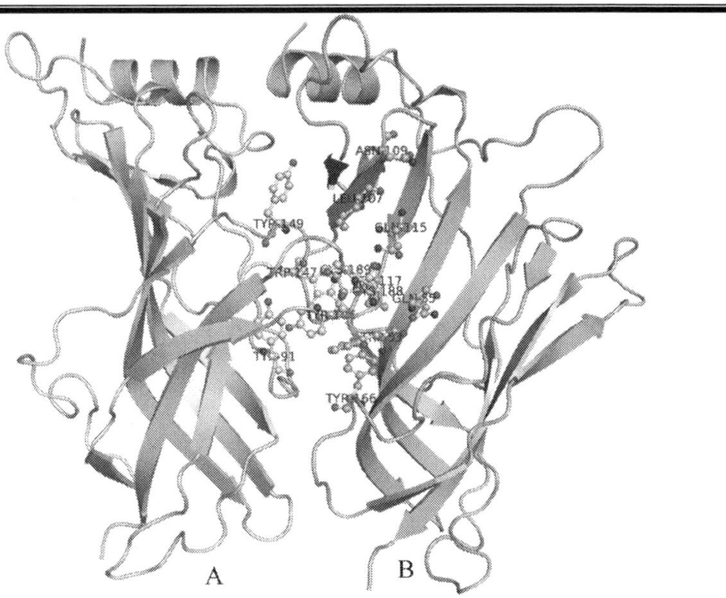

Figure 12: Represenatation of the residues at the interface region on a schematic secondary structure. The figure shows the plus face of the subunit A (light cyan color) and the minus face of the subunit B (light pink). The interface residues were represented in ball and stick representation. The actual interaction may vary in LGIC interface, but in all receptors these topological regions were likely to form the interface.

109, GLN 115, LEU 117), loop F (TYR 166) respectively [Fig. 12]. The disulphide bridge is present only in the alpha subunit of nAChR and is known to be a part of agonist binding site of the receptor. Both the subunits contribute residues for ligand binding effectively. From this, it is clear that the dimer interface region includes the ligand binding pocket, which possesses a disulfide bridge containing loop C. In order to explore the binding properties of this cleft, the theoretical model is pointed to docking experiments were carried out for the model in future.

The steps taken earlier by researchers, for the construction of the theoretical model to study the nAChRs were in different class and subunits of muscle type of nAChR (Konstantakaki *et al.* 2007). The Homology modeling approach was even applied to the Transmembrane helices of various subunits to know about the channel gating process (Arias *et al.* 2001). In particular a theoretical model of Extracellular domain of human α_7nAChR was also reported based on the crystal structure solved at 1.94Å resolution of mouse α_1nAChR extracellular domain of muscle type complexed with α-bungarotoxin (Konstantakaki *et al.* 2008). Due to this complex nature in the crystal structure of mouse α_1nAChR, the Cys loop remains to be in open state when compared with other small ligand bound complex (Brejc *et al.* 2001), and thus we neglected this structure usage. To our knowledge this is the first attempt to reveal the mystery behind the structural aspects of human α_7nAChR. With this information researchers will find it easy to narrow down the path towards rationalized drug design by 3D-Quantitative Structure Activity Relationship (3D-QSAR), Combinatorial Chemistry, High Throughput Screening (HTS) approaches. The lead molecule generated by these computational approaches were expected to drastically reduces the time duration, money, manpower which is usually the longest and most expensive stage in the drug discovery process.

2. Molecular interaction of agonist and competitive antagonist with Human Neuronal α_7nAChR.

The theoretical structure of nAChR

The theoretical structure of the nAChR were constructed using homology modelling approach which uses the structural template from *Lymnea stagnalis* which shares good structural similarity. The theoretical structure was subjected to reduce the geometic inaccuracies and analysed using series of steps to make the structure usable for the further investigations. This structure generated from our previous study and was used for our current docking and interaction studies [15].

α-BTX:

Molecular docking studies between theoretical model of nAChR and the snake three fingered α-BTX of long α-neurotoxin were performed. This interaction study helps us in understanding the binding mode of the ligands and also to validate the generated theoretical model. α-BTX, which is a α-neurotoxin, acts as a competitive inhibitor and blocks α_7nAChR [Fig.13]. The α-BTX is the member of three-fingered long α-neurotoxins comprising of two antiparallel β sheets. The α-BTX posses three loops, loop I-III, that emerge from the dense core containing 5 disulphide bridges. It forms a slightly concave disk elongated in the direction of the long loop II that bears ASP 30, VAL 31, PHE 32, CYS 33, SER 34, SER 35, ARG 36 and GLY 37 respectively. The α-neurotoxin is principally characterized by the fifth disulphide bond. The loop II seems to insert deeply into the ligand binding pocket located at the interface, between nAChR subunit.

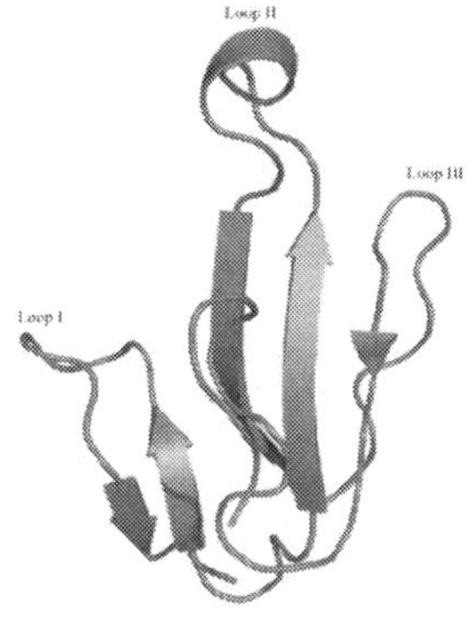

Figure 13: Experimental structure of monomer α-BTX (PDB code: 1HC9) with continuous β sheet and three loops. The α helix present at the loopII fits around the receptor binding site loop and in addition binds tightly at the interface of the two of the receptor subunits.

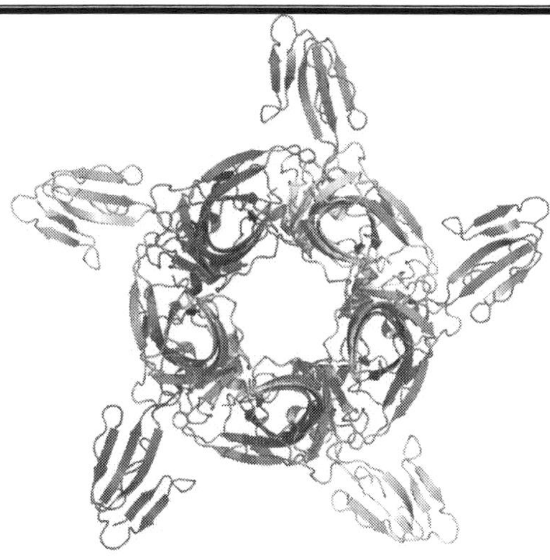

Figure 14: Overall view of α_7nAChR- α-BTX complex viewed along 5-fold axis of the pentamer. The toxin inserts a finger perpendicularly to the α_7nAChR pentamer.

Interaction between nAChR – α-BTX:

The program 3D-Dock was used for docking of α-BTX with the theoretical structure of nAChR which allows an exhaustive search on theoretical nAChR for binding interface. The nAChR - α-BTX complex was generated by rigid body docking procedure. The nAChR - α-BTX complex reveals that the toxin is tightly bound at the binding pocket of the theoretical model, such that the loop II of the toxin properly penetrates at the interface region of theoretical nAChR [Fig.14].

On the other hand, numerous clashes were observed between nAChR - α-BTX at the subunit interface carrying the complementary component of the binding site. Energy minimization procedure with 100 iterations was done using SYBYL to remove bumps & steric clashes. The resulting complex was further investigated in terms of buried surface area and number of

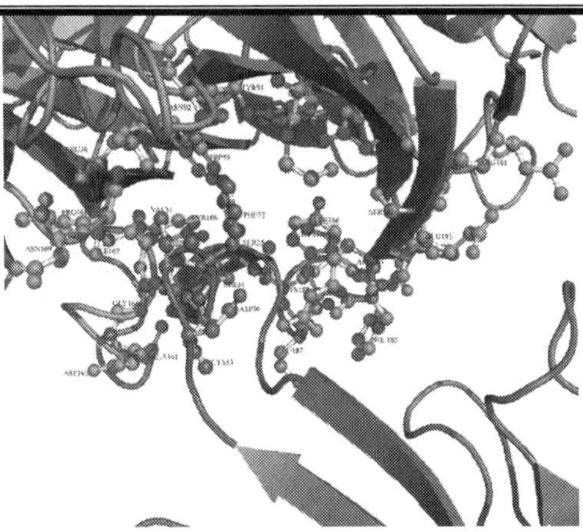

Figure 15: Close view of the model α_7nAChR pentamer bound to toxin at single interface. The toxin inserts fingerII which shares ASP 30, VAL 31, PHE 32, CYS 33, SER 34, SER 35, ARG 36, and GLY 37 with nAChR subunit at interfaces.

residues involved in interactions [Fig.15]. It was clearly observed that the binding pocket was dominated by aromatic and hydrophobic residues at the cleft region. In the principle chain of nAChR, Cys-188 was found in proximity with SER 35 and ARG 36 with TYR 186. On the complementary side ASP 162 interacts with CYS 33, ALA 161 with SER 34 and TYR 166 with SER 35.

The theoretical model of nAChR, α-BTX and the nAChR - α-BTX complexes were individually subjected to the online web interface VADAR for the investigation of Accessible Surface Area (ASA). The results produced by VADAR between bound and unbound complexes were compared and the residues involved in binding of nAChR - α-BTX complex tabulated [Table 5]. The drastic reduction in the surface area of the residues which are involved in the binding of nAChR- α-BTX complex was clearly observed at the antagonist binding site. Moreover, the interactions of the nAChR-α-BTX complex at the interface region were investigated by subjecting it to protein-protein interaction server. This result yielded the list of residues which are involved in the ligand binding site [Table 6]; of which majority of the residues coincide with the results form VADAR server. Subsequently, the complex was submitted to the online web interface WhatIf to determine the potential Hydrogen bonds interactions between nAChR-α-BTX complexes. The H-bonds between the residues of bound complex [Table 7] were investigated by DEEP-VIEW (Kaplan and Littlejohn 2001) and residues involved in the interaction were in concurrence with previous results. By this, it is apparent that homomeric receptors recognize this toxin at the interface regions. This observation could shed new light in understanding of the strong α-BTX binding to nAChR.

Table 5: Volume Angle Dihedral Angle Report (VADAR). Accessible Surface Area calculated for residues involved in nAChR-α-BTX binding is compared with bound and unbound complexes. The result was produced using online server VADAR.

A-Chain (nAChR)	RESIDUES		ASA Before docking	ASA After docking
1	185	PHE	101.5	15.2
2	186	TYR	54.5	12.8
3	187	GLU	160.9	140.7
4	188	CYS	104.7	93.6
5	189	CYS	35.7	26.6
B-Chain (nAChR)				
1	33	LEU	14.5	10.9
2	34	SER	14.8	8.0
3	161	ALA	66.1	54.8
4	162	ASP	87.1	55.8
5	163	ILE	47.2	44.9
6	164	SER	44.8	40.6
7	165	GLY	50.4	1.2
8	166	TYR	82.3	16.5
9	167	ILE	18.8	15.1
Toxin (α-BTX)				
1	30	ASP	63.8	51.7
2	31	VAL	130.8	42.3
3	32	PHE	93.3	6.5
4	33	CYS	26.9	8.5
5	34	SER	117.8	14.1
6	35	SER	96.2	6.5
7	36	ARG	166.6	7.8
8	37	GLY	39.8	13.9

Table 6: Results from Protein-Protein interaction server (PPI). Key residues involved in nAChR-α-BTX binding were retrieved from Protein-Protein interaction server.

A-Chain (nAChR)		B-Chain (nAChR)		TOXIN (α-BTX)	
91	TYR	36	LEU	29	CYS
92	ASN	53	TRP	30	ASP
143	LYS	161	ALA	31	VAL
181	ARG	162	ASP	32	PHE
182	SER	165	GLY	33	CYS
183	GLU	166	TYR	34	SER
184	ARG	167	ILE	35	SER
185	PHE	168	PRO		
186	TYR	169	ASN		
187	GLU				
188	CYS				
189	CYS				
190	LYS				
192	PRO				
195	ASP				

Table 7: Hydrogen bond calculation. Potential hydrogen bonds between residues involved in nAChR-αBTX binding. The results were obtained from online WhatIf servers.

S.No	(+)chain(nAChR)		(α-BTX)	
1	184	ARG	30	ASP
2	184	ARG	30	ASP
3	184	ARG	32	PHE
4	187	GLU	35	SER
5	188	CYS	35	SER
	(-)Chain (nAChR)		(α-BTX)	
6	34	SER	34	SER
7	166	TYR	35	SER
8	166	TYR	35	SER
9	166	TYR	36	ARG

Interaction between nAChR – agonists (Acetylcholine and Nicotine):

The small molecule ligands Acetylcholine and Nicotine [Fig. 16] were obtained from PubChem database for docking with theoretical nAChR pentamer. The pentameric nAChR was prepared by

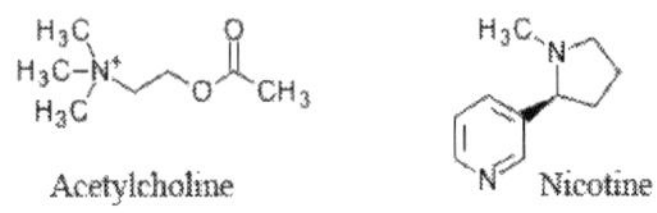

Figure 16: The chemical structure of Acetylcholine and Nicotine reterieved form PubChem Database.

assigning potentials. The small molecules were prepared by assigning formal charge of +1. The powerful approach of flexible docking for nAChR-agonists was performed using AUTODOCK3. The program AutoDock provides an automated procedure for predicting the interaction of ligands with bio-macromolecular targets which applies Monte Carlo (MC) and Simulated Annealing (SA) technique using grid-based molecular affinity potentials. The grid was generated arbitrarily at the interface of the theoretical model nAChR. Up to 50 docking procedures were run for each ligand which subsequently produced 4 to 10 clusters. Based on the highest size among the clusters produced, only one docking was selected for each ligand, which was found to be common for the two ligands [Fig.17].

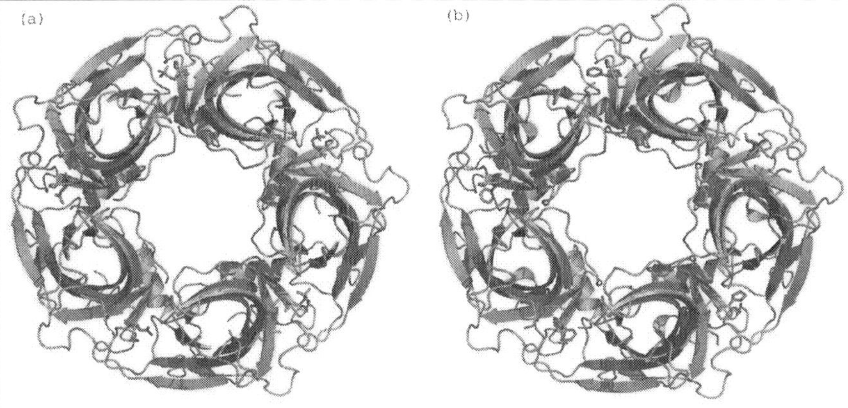

Figure 17: Full View of the pentamer model docked with (a) acetylcholine and (b) nicotine at 5 interfaces.

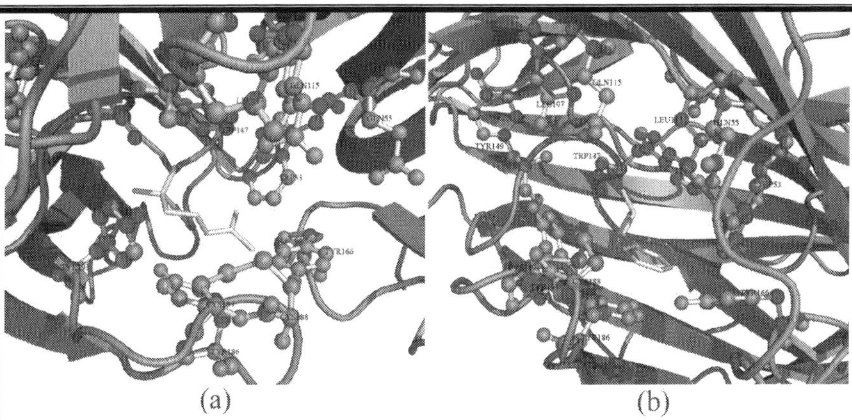

Figure 18: Close view of pentamer docked with (a) acetylcholine and (b) nicotine at single interface. The agonist molecules buried well in aromatic and hydrophobic cleft are seen clearly.

The functional gorge of the receptor molecule was contributed by both (+) side and (–) side chains for agonists binding effectively. This core was dominated by aromatic and hydrophobic residues which contribute TYR 91, TRP 147, TYR 149, TYR 186, CYS 188, CYS 189, and TYR 193 from principle side and the complementary side residues from TRP 53, GLU 55, LEU 107, ASN 109, GLN 115, LEU 117, and TYR 166 resulting in efficient docking. [Fig.18].

However, because of the uncertainty on the comparative modeling process and the sequence identity shared between template and the target of about 22.4%, it is pointed out that absolute values are to be considered with caution at this stage.

A dimer of nAChR-agonists was examined using an online web server LIGPLOT where the protein ligand interactions were schematically represented [Fig.19]. Subsequently, the docked complexes were analyzed by subjecting the complex to online web server Ligand Protein Contact (LPC). The output yielded the residues [Table 8 and 9] which are in contact with the agonists out of which majority of the residues were found to be similar to the Ligplot results. The residues which contact the agonist's molecule are shown in Figure 19.

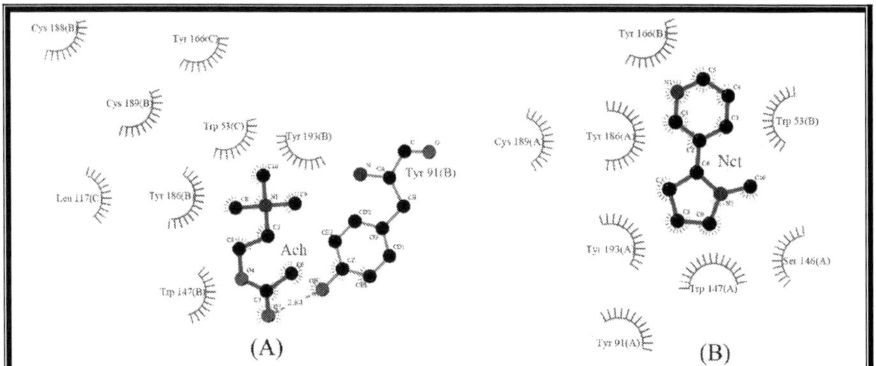

Figure 19: Ligplot results display the (a) acetylcholine and (b) nicotine buried in aromatic and hydrophobic cleft. Schematic ligand interaction of acetylcholine showing hydrogen bond to the hydroxyl group of TYR 91 and both (a) acetylcholine and (b) nicotine buried well inside hydrophobic and aromatic cleft is seen clearly.

By this it is clear that ligands are buried at hydrophobic and aromatic binding pocket of human α_7nAChR.

Table 8: Ligand protein interaction. The key residues involved in nAChR-acetylcholine binding were retrieved form LPC-CSU server. Majority of the residues which bind to ligand are hydrophobic.

S.No	Residue		Specific contacts		
			HB	Arom	Phob
1	91A	TYR*	-	-	-
2	146A	SER	-	-	-
3	147A	TRP*	-	-	-
4	186A	TYR*	-	-	+
5	188A	CYS*	-	-	-
6	189A	CYS*	-	-	-
7	193A	TYR*	-	-	-
8	53B	TRP*	+	-	+
9	117B	LEU*	-	-	+
10	166B	TYR*	-	-	+

Table 9: Ligand protein interaction. The key residues involved in nAChR-nicotine binding were retrieved form LPC-CSU server.

S.No	Residue		Specific contacts		
			HB	Arom	Phob
1	91A	TYR*	-	+	-
2	146A	SER	-	-	-
3	147A	TRP*	+	+	-
4	148A	SER*	-	-	-
5	186A	TYR*	-	+	+
6	188A	CYS*	-	-	-
7	189A	CYS*	-	-	-
8	193A	TYR*	-	+	+
9	53B	TRP*	-	+	-
10	107B	LEU*	-	-	-
11	117B	LEU*	-	-	+
12	166B	TYR*	-	+	-

HB – Hydrophilic contact
Arom - Aromatic contact
Phob - Hydrophobic contact

As mentioned earlier, a theoretical model of Extracellular domain of human α_7nAChR was also reported based on the crystal structure solved at 1.94Å resolution of mouse α_1nAChR extracellular domain of muscle type complexed with α-bungarotoxin (Konstantakaki *et al.* 2008). The work reported by us in addition to studying the interactions of acetylcholine with the pentameric receptor also includes the study of interactions of additional ligands, nicotine and α-bungarotoxin with this model. Another molecular docking studies relating to α-cobratoxin (Konstantakaki *et al.* 2007) and α-conotoxin (Adams *et al.* 2003; Nicke *et al.* 2003; Armishaw *et al.* 2009) with nAChR also supports our study, i.e., the binding site residues of nAChRs which is proposed by us is coinciding with other docking results. In the case of cobra toxin the third loop which is finger shaped properly gets inserted into interface region.

3. *Insilico* Point mutations and Evolutionary Trace Analysis applied to Human Neuronal α_7nAChR.

Theoretical model

In our previous studies, the theoretical model of α_7nAChR was performed in detail. The studies involved retrieval of the sequence of LBD of α_7nAChR from SwissProt and submitted to NCBI-Blast and PSIPRED to get the homologues template. This gives out the crystal structure of AChBP (PDB ID: 1I9B) of snail as the structural template which is refined at 2.7Å resolution. The sequence of α_7nAChR shares about 22.4% identity with the template and was aligned using EBI-align. Moreover there was good agreement between the secondary structural elements of both sequences in the crucial regions. The alignment was further improved by JalView, a java based alignment editor. This alignment was used for construction of the theoretical structure of α_7nAChR using Modeller9v2. The Modeller9v2 produces 20 individual models, out of which only one representative structure with minimum energy was selected. Based on the initial equivalencies from EBI-Dalilite server the theoretical subunit was assembled into pentamer using InsightII and subsequently minimized using Sybyl7.1 up to 100 iterations to remove the steric clashes at the interfaces. The theoretical structure was examined for Structurally Variable Region (SVRs) and Structurally Conserved Regions (SCRs). This exhibits similar regions with that of AChBP with that of α_7nAChR [Fig. 20a & 20b]. The electrostatic potential map from PyMol exhibits the channel is highly cationic in nature [Fig. 21]. With this template molecular docking studies was performed with a cluster of small molecule which is agonists and antagonists in its nature (Parthiban *et al.* 2009).

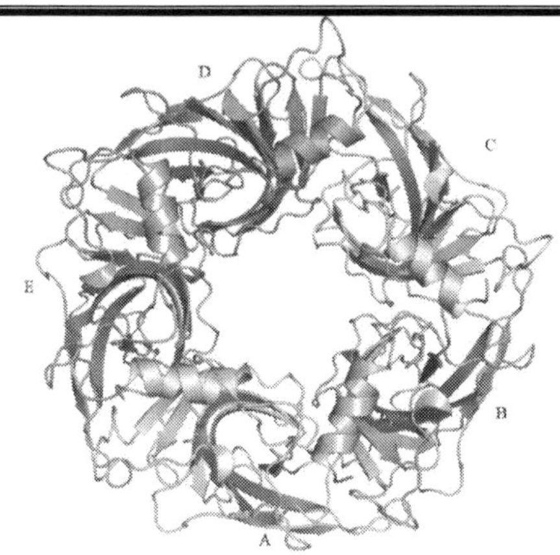

Figure 20a

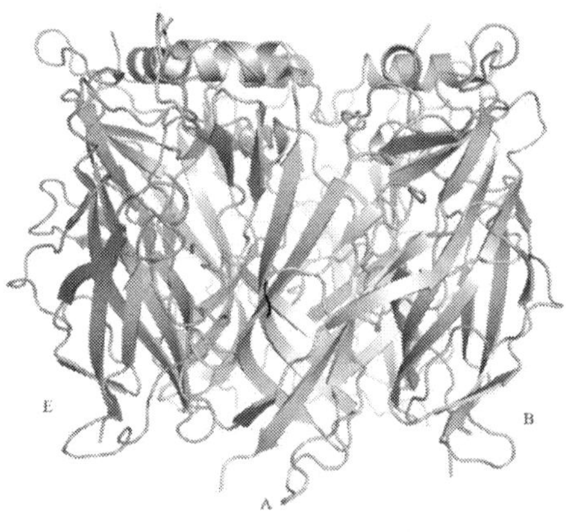

Figure20b

The theoretical model of pentameric human α_7 nAChR. (1a) In this representation, each subunit is displayed in different color. The subunits were labeled anti-clockwise, with A-B, B-C, C-D, D-E and E-A forming the + and – chain. This forms the principle and the complementary ligand binding sites, respectively. (1b) displays the nAChR pentamer perpendicular to the fivefold axis. The ligand binding sites were located equatorially and are highlighted in different colors.

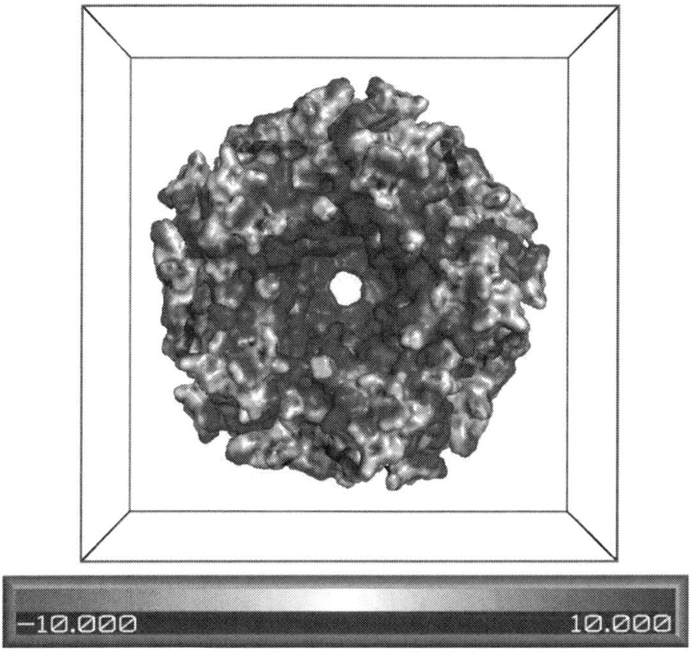

Figure 21: The electrostatic potential map showing the interior of the pentameric α_7nAChR is highly negative. The potential map was rendered using PyMol.

Ligand Preparation (Agonist and Antagonist) and Processing for Molecular Docking with α_7nAChR model

All the small molecules which is said to be agonist and antagonists were retrieved from PUBCHEM database [Fig. 22]. These molecules were obtained in the form of 2D from the database. These ligand molecules were further processed by converting into 3D coordinates by VLife MDS Suite. These 3D coordinates of agonists and antagonists molecules were further processed by subjecting them to energy minimization by applying MMCF force field for up to 100 iterations, in order to bring the ligand molecules to lower energy and away from the structural clashes which will best suits for docking studies. These processed molecules were used for protein-ligand docking studies in further.

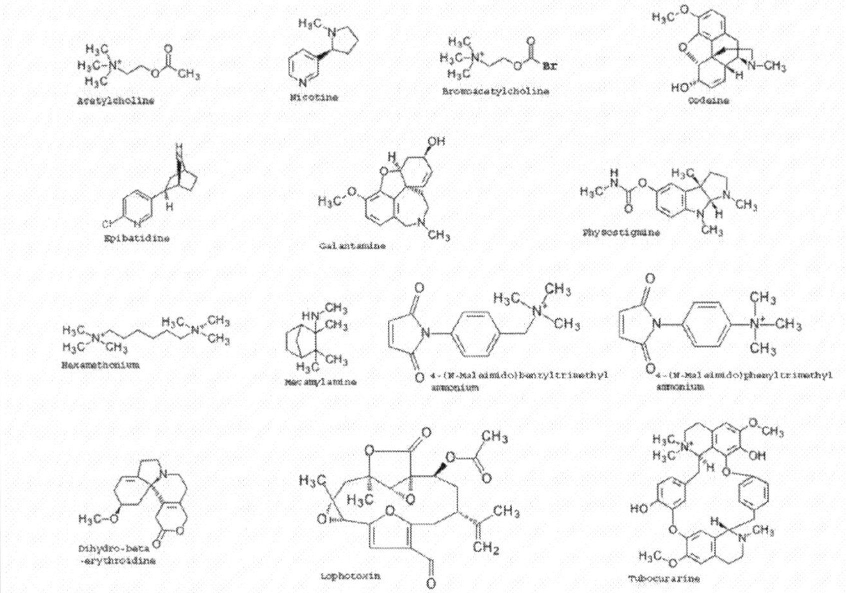

Figure 22: List of ligands which is grouped as agonists and antagonists used for the docking studies with the theoretical model of α_7nAChR.

Protein-Ligand docking studies on α_7nAChR

A typical docking study was carried out on the theoretical structure of α_7nAChR from our previous studies with its agonists and antagonists. The selected structure of α_7nAChR was effectively represented as an energetically favorable conformational structure after a series of analysis tools. AutoDock4.0 was used for the docking study which is an automated molecular docking software package, which offers a variety of search algorithms to explore a given docking problem. This includes Monte Carlo Simulated Annealing (SA); a Genetic Algorithm (GA); and a hybrid local search GA, also known as the Lamarckian Genetic Algorithm (LGA).

Since α_7nAChR is a homopentamer, this pentamer is reduced to homodimer for docking experiments for consistency, and is believed that this binding is common for all five binding site. The docking was tried to perform "protein and flexible-ligand" and "protein and rigid-ligand" docking studies to enhance the sampling space of protein ligand interactions [Table 10a & 10b]. In the case of flexible-ligand interactions the torsion angles of the ligands were allowed to rotate freely and on the other hand rigid ligand interaction the torsion angle of the ligands were kept rigid. By specifying the locations of the binding site, significantly narrow down the search time. AutoDock provides an automated procedure for predicting the interaction of ligands with bio-molecular targets in which Genetic Algorithm (GA) technique is applied using grid-based molecular affinity potentials. Thus grid is positioned at -14.699Å x -26.356Å x -3.099Å arbitrarily i.e. between the interface region of the theoretical structure of α_7nAChR which is supposed to be the active site of the receptor, and also by providing the rotation space of about 0.536Å, the docking calculations were carried out for 100 cycles for all the ligands respectively.

The outputs form the docking of 100 GA runs was ranked according to the binding energy and clustering histogram. The scoring functions is based on the energy terms, namely, protein-ligand Van der Waals energy, distance between the interacting atoms, dissolving energy, electrostatic energy, torsion free energy and unbound system's energy. AutoDock has an inbuilt clustering method based on the RMSD values, which is used for clustering the ligand poses having the clustering RMSD of >0.04Å. According to the binding energy, the top scoring energy ligand orientations are considered as the best ligand poses [Fig. 23a & 23b]. By considering the higher number of cluster formation and the best binding energy the protein-ligand complexes were collected as the final docking result for all the ligands respectively [Table 11].

These complexes were analyzed for bonded and the non-bonded interactions using AutoDock inbuilt modules and with our in-house program Interactor. The functional gorge of the receptor molecule was contributed by both (+) side and (-) side chains for agonists binding effectively. In the docking analysis most of the small molecules were found to interact with the cysteine residue (188-189) at the binding pocket and is dominated by hydrophobic and aromatic residues form the (+) side domain. The efficient docking analysis reports, that this core was dominated by aromatic and hydrophobic residues which contribute TYR91, TRP147, TYR149, TYR186, CYS188-189

TABLE 10A: Neuronal α_7nAChR interacts with agonist molecule.

S.No	Ligand	Energy Kcal/Mol	Interacting Residues
1	**Acetylcholine**	-3.58	TYR91, SER146, TRP147, TYR186, CYS188, CYS189, TYR193, TRP53, LEU117
2	**Nicotine**	-4.13	TYR91, SER146, TRP147, SER148, TYR 186, CYS188, CYS189, TYR193, TRP53, LEU107, LEU117, TYR116
3	**Acetylcholine Mustard**	-2.47	CYS189, TYR166, SER34, LEU117, TRP53, TRP147
4	**Bromoacetylcholine**	-4.09	GLN115, LEU117, TRP147, TYR193, CYS189, LYS190
5	**Carbamylcholine**	-0.99	TRP147, LEU107, LEU117, GLN115, CYS188, CYS189
6	**Codeine**	-4.27	CYS188, LYS190, HIS113, ASN109, VAL108, LEU107
7	**Epibatidine**	-4.81	TRP147, TYR186, CYS188, CYS189, TYR166, GLN115, LEU117, LEU109
8	**Cyticine**	-5.86	TRP53, LEU117, TRP147, TYR166, CYS189
9	**Galanthamide**	-4.63	ASN109, HIS113, LEU107, LYS190, THR75, GLN115
10	**Physostigmine**	-3.85	ALA161, TYR166, TYR86, ARG184, GLY187

Table 10B: Neuronal α_7nAChR interacts with antagonist molecule

S.No	Ligand	Energy Kcal/Mol	Interacting Residues
11	**Hexamethonium**	-4.35	CYS189,TYR193, TRP143, TRP53, LEY117, GLN115, LEU107
12	**Serotonin**	-3.92	TRP117, CYS189, CYS188, TYR166, GLU115, LEU107, TRP53, SER34
13	**Mecamylamine**	-4.35	CYS188, CYS189, TYR193, TRP147, LEU117, GLU115, LEU107
14	**4-(N-Maleimido)benzyltrimethylammonium**	-6.99	CYS188, CYS189, GLU55, TYR166, LEU117, GLN115, LEU 107, TRP147
15	**4-(N-Maleimido)phenyltrimethylammonium**	-6.64	CYS188, CYS189, GLN55, GLU115, LEU107, SER148, TRP147, LEU117, SER34, TYR166
16	**Phencyclidine**	-6.07	CYS188, CYS189, TYR193, TRP147, LEU117, GLN115
17	**dihydro-beta-erythroiodine**	-3.70	TYR147, TYR186, CYS188, CYS 189, TYR166, GLNM115, LEU117, LEU109
18	**Lophotoxin**	-5.86	HIS113, ASN 109, THR75, LYS118, LYS190, SER148
19	**d-tubocurarine**	-6.92	THR75, GLN115, LEU107, LYS74, HIS113, PHE185, LYS190, LYS74, CYS188, CYS190, GLU189

Table 10A & 10B displays the docking of α_7 nAChR with the ligand agonists and antagonists respectively. The docking was performed using Autodock4.0. The energy calculations and the interacting residues were picked out using the inbuilt module in AutoDock 4.0.

Table 11: Rigid ligand interaction

S.No	Agonist	Energy Kcal/Mol	Interacting residues
1	**Bromoacetylcholine**	-6.34	**SER34**, TRP53, LET117, **TYR116,** TYR186,CYS188
2	**Nicotine**	-9.11	**LEU107**, TRP147, TYR186, CYS189, TYR193
3	**Codeine**	-10.40	TRP53, **LEY107, GLN115,** LEU117, TRP147, **SER148,** CYS188, CYS189, TYR193
4	**Epibatidine**	-9.46	**TRP53, LEU117**, SER146, TRP147, **TYR186, CYS188, CYS189, TYR193**
5	**Galanthamine**	-10.56	LEU107, LEU117, **TRP147**, SER148, **TYR186, CYS188, CYS189, TYR193**
	Antagonist		
6	**Hexamethionium**	-6.25	**TRP53**, LEU107, **TRP147**, TYR166, **TYR186, CYS189, TYR193**
7	**Mecalamine**	-10.08	**TRP53, LEU117, TRP147, TYR186, CYS189, TYR193**
8	**4-(N-Maleimido)benzyltrimethylammonium**	-8.37	GLN55, GLN115, **LEU117, TYR186, CYS186, CYS188, CYS189, TYR193**
9	**4-(N-Maleimido)phenyltrimethylammonium**	-8.93	SER34, **TRP53**, GLN55, **TRP147**, TYR166, **CYS188, TYR193**
10	**dihydro-beta-erythroiodine**	-9.47	**TRP53**, LEU107, GLN115, **LEU117, TRP147, CYS188, CYS189, TYR193**
11	**Lophotoxin**	-8.36	**TRP53**, LEU107, GLN115, **LEU117, TRP147**, SER148, TYR166, **CYS188, CYS189, TYR193**
12	**d-tubocurarine**	-7.84	GLN55, LEU107, ASN109, HIS113, GLN115, **LEU117**, GLN157, **CYS188, CYS189**, LYS190, **TYR193**

The ligands which show the best binding energies from pervious docking were alone selected and again docking was performed by reducing torsion (rigid) of the ligand to zero. The key residues which are found to interact with nAChRs were conserved and are highlighted. Most of the residues are hydrophobic. The binding energy found to be very good than the earlier.

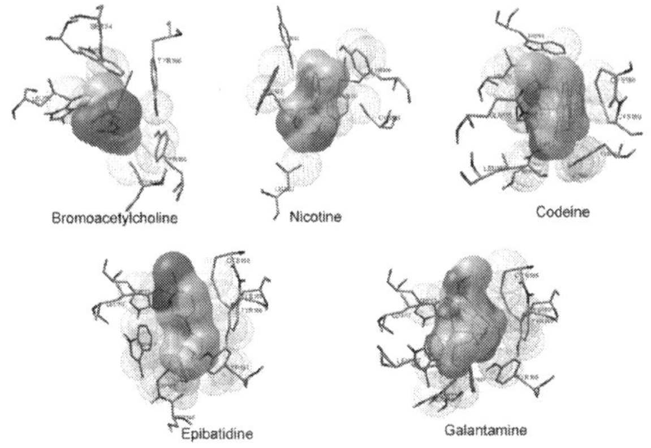

Figure 23a

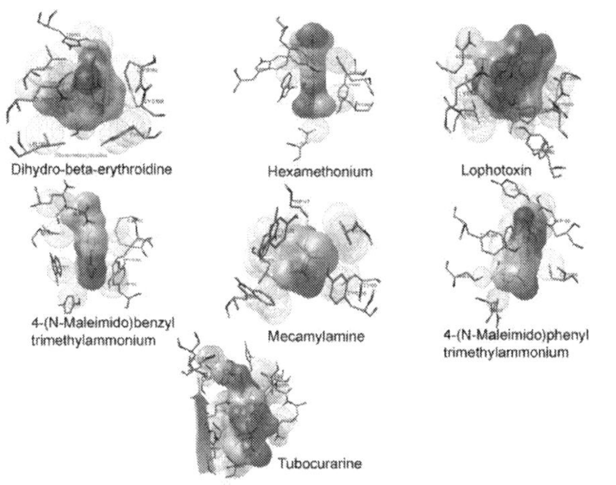

Figure 23b

Rigid ligand interaction with α_7nAChR. 4A shows the agonists interact with the α_7nAChR. 4B shows the antagonists with interacts with α_7nAChR. The interactions were obtained from the inbuilt module from AutoDock.

Figure 24: Point Mutation on α_7nAChR

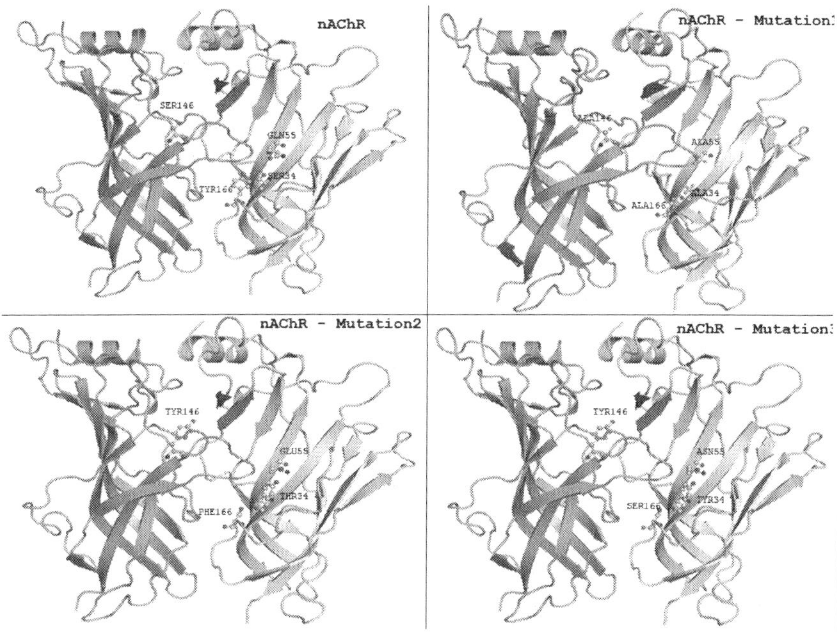

The theoretical models were subjected to mutation based on the interaction of class-specific residues. This mutation is of three types and the residues were mutated based on the residual property.

The protein-rigid ligand interaction shows best binding energy with good in number of clusters formation than the protein-flexible ligand interaction which is preferred for the analysis and further study. The ligands which show very less binding energy and improper cluster formations were neglected, because of unable to infer information out of the interactions. The new residues which appear in the interaction result were mapped on the alignment of the α_7nAChR and its close homologue. These new residues were SER146 (+), SER34 (-), GLN55 (-) and TYR166 (-) was aimed to concentrate to explore more about the conserved and class-specific residues among the α_7nAChR homologues [Fig. 24]. These new residues were then mutated to three different approaches based on the property of the residue involved. The SER146 of (+) chain was mutated to ALA, THR and TYR; SER34 of (-) chain was replaced by ALA, THR and TYR; GLN55 of (-) chain was substituted to ALA, GLU and ASN; and finally TYR166 of (-) chain was mutated to ALA, PHE and SER respectively using SYBYL7.1. These three mutated theoretical α_7nAChR was subsequently energy minimized to reduce the steric clashes and geometric inaccuracies occurred due to induced point residue mutation using TRIPOS force field. This reduces distorted energy occurred due to point residue mutation in the α_7nAChR to global minimal energy state, which was represented as energetically well stable and favorable structure for analysis. To our knowledge, it is apparent that this type of Insilico point mutational investigations was not performed earlier.

Protein-Ligand docking studies on point residue mutation on α_7nAChR

The docking was carried out for these three different mutated α_7nAChR structures by applying the same procedure by keeping the ligand as rigid for 100 cycles. The docking produces clusters of ligand interacting with α_7nAChR with high binding energy. The three different mutation induced structure of α_7nAChR docked with the rigid ligands was subjected to analysis for interacting residues in AutoDock separately.

Mutation 1:

In the first type of mutation all the newly interacting residues were replaced by ALA to test the occurrences of ALA is all the subsequent rigid docking with the ligands. The docking complexes were analyzed for interacting residues with the ligands using AUTODOCK [Fig 25a & 25b]. Since ALA possesses the smaller side chain, this residue appeared in very few docking complexes [Table 12]. The docking complexes were subjected to H-bond analysis using the in-house program Interactor. This program strips out the residue which has hydrogen bond interaction with the ligands. In this analysis, there is no H-bond formation is observed with the ligand and receptor [Table 15]. The docking result turns out to be less effective with the binding energy and the cluster formation. By this, it is suggested that this docking is not that much effective in binding with ligands.

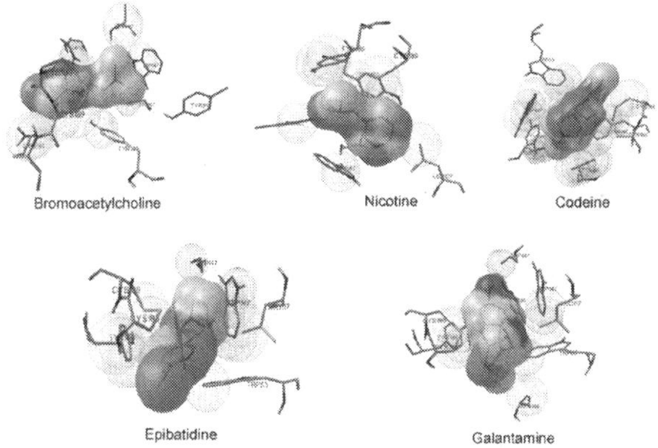

Figure 25a

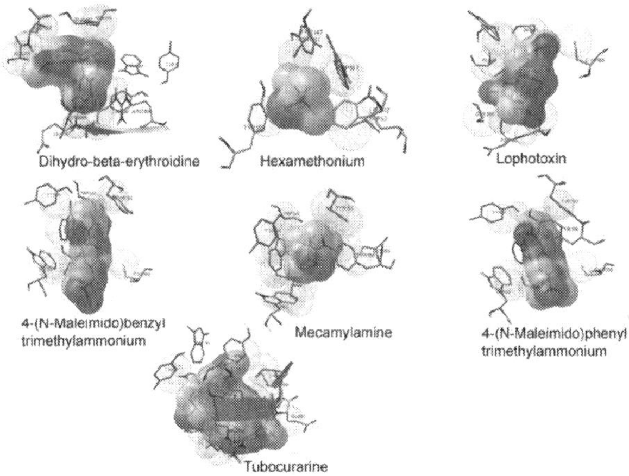

Figure 25b

Rigid ligand interaction with mutated α_7nAChR. 6a shows the agonists interacts with the mutated α_7nAChR. 6b shows the antagonists with interacts with mutated α_7nAChR. The interactions were obtained from the inbuilt module from AutoDock.

Table 12: Mutation 01

S.No	Agonist	Energy Kcal/Mol	Interacting residues
1	**Bromoacetylcholine**	-6.12	GLN115,LEU117,TRP147,CYS188,CYS189,LYS190,TYR193
2	**Nicotine**	-8.98	LEU107,TRP147,TYR186,CYS189,TYR193
3	**Codeine**	-10.40	TRP53, TYR186,TRP147,CYS188,CYS189,TYR193
4	**Epibatidine**	-9.36	TRP53,LEU117,TRP147,TYR186,CYS188,CYS189
5	**Galanthamine**	-9.36	TRP53,LEU107,GLN115,LEU117,TRP147,CYS188,CYS189,TYR193
	Antagonist		
6	**Hexamethionium**	-6.03	TRP53,TYR147,TYR186,CYS189,TYR193
7	**Mecalamine**	-9.87	TRP53,LEU117,TRP147,TYR186,CYS189,TYR193
8	**4-(N-Maleimido)benzyltrimethylammonium**	-8.03	TRP53,LEU117,TRP147,CYS188,TYR193
9	**4-(N-Maleimido)phenyltrimethylammonium**	-8.35	TRP53,LEU117,TRP147,TYR186,CYS188,TYR193
10	**dihydro-beta-erythroiodine**	-8.84	LEU107,ASN109,HIS113,GLN115,CYS188,LYS190
11	**Lophotoxin**	-10.73	SER32,**ALA34**,TRP53,**ALA55**,ALA161,ASP162,GLY165,CYS188
12	**d-tubocurarine**	-9.72	TRP53,ALA161,**ALA166**,GLY165,ARG184,TYR186,GLU187,CYS188,CYS189,TYR193

The class-specific residues which were identified using docking were subjected to mutation type 1. The mutation involves the substitution of SER146 (+), SER34 (-), GLN55 (-) and TYR166 (-) with ALA using Sybyl 7.1. The occurances of mutated residues were highlighted.

Mutation 2:

In the second type of mutation SER146 (+) chain was replaced with THR, SER34 (-) was replaced with THR, GLN55 (-) was replaced with GLU and TYR166 (-) was replaced with PHE. The docking result turns out with good binding energy and with good cluster formation when compared with the first type of mutation. When the complexes were analyzed for interaction using AUTODOCK [Fig 26a & 26b], GLU55 occurs in many cases of interaction and CYS 188-189 was found to occur in all the cases [Table 13]. The docking complexes were subjected to our in-house program Interactor, which particularly displays the H-bond interacting residues. This displays GLU55 which has H-bond interaction with the ligand molecule [Table 15]. By this, it clarifies the result that this docking is pretty effective to binding with ligands.

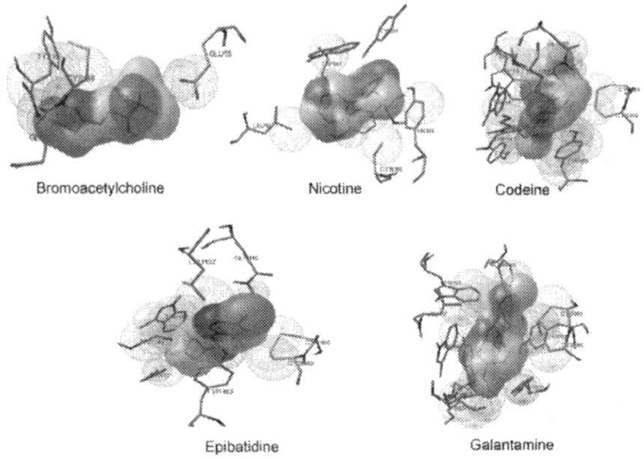

Figure 26a

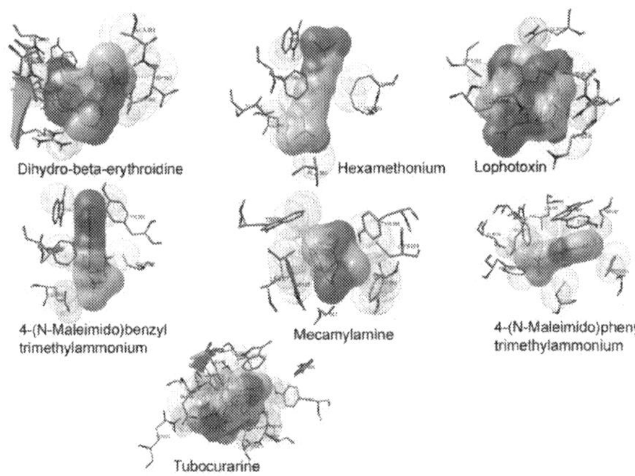

Figure 26b

Rigid ligand interaction with mutated α_7nAChR. 7a shows the agonists interacts with the mutated α_7nAChR. 7b shows the antagonists with interacts with mutated α_7nAChR. The interactions were obtained from the inbuilt module from AutoDock.

Table 13: Mutation 02

S.No	Agonist	Energy Kcal/Mol	Interacting residues
1	**Bromoacetylcholine**	-6.78	**GLU55**,PHE166,TYR186,GLU187,CYS188
2	**Nicotine**	-9.14	LEU107,TRP147,TYR186,CYS189,TYR193
3	**Codeine**	-10.36	TRP53,LEU107,GLN115,LEU117,TRP147,SER148, CYS188,CYS189,TYR193
4	**Epibatidine**	-9.43	TRP53,PHE116,LEU117,**THR146**,TRP147,TYR186, CYS188,CYS189,TYR193
5	**Galanthamine**	-10.62	TRP53,LEU107,LEU117,TRP147,SER148,TYR186,CYS188,CYS189,TYR193
	Antagonist		
6	**Hexamethionium**	-6.71	**GLU55**,PHE166,TYR186,CYS188,CYS189,TYR193
7	**Mecalamine**	-10.19	TRP53,TRP147,TYR186,CYS189,TYR193
8	**4-(N-Maleimido)benzyltrimethylammonium**	-9.00	**GLU55**,GLN115,LEU117,PHE166,TYR186,CYS188
9	**4-(N-Maleimido)phenyltrimethylammonium**	-9.36	**GLU55**,LEU117,PHE166,TYR186,CYS188
10	**dihydro-beta-erythroiodine**	-9.06	ALA161,ASP162,GLY165,TYR166,ARG184,TYR186,GLU187,CYS188
11	**Lophotoxin**	-9.54	LYS74,THR75,LEU107,ASN109,GLN115,CYS188,CYS189,LYS190,TYR193
12	**d-tubocurarine**	-4.80	**GLU55**,LEU107,ASN109,HIS113,GLN115,LEU117,CYS188,CYS189,LYS190,TYR193

The class-specific residues which were identified using docking were subjected to mutation type 2. The mutation involves the substitution of SER146 (+) with THR, SER34 (-) with THR, GLN55 (-) with GLU and TYR166 (-) with PHE respectively using Sybyl 7.1. The occurances of mutated residues were highlighted.

Mutation 3:

In the third type of mutation SER146 (+) chain was replaced with TYR, SER34 (-) was replaced with TYR, GLN55 (-) was replaced with ASN and TYR166 (-) was replaced with SER. The docking result turns out with good binding energy and with good cluster formation when compared with the rest of the two types of mutation. The complexes were subsequently subjected to analyze the interacting residues using AUTODOCK [Fig. 27a & 27b]. SER166 and TYR146 appear in many of the cases of antagonists. Also the CYS 188-189 was found to occur in all the cases [Table 14]. When the docked complexes were subjected to Interactor, the H-bond interaction was displayed with TYR146 and SER166 in few cases [Table 15]. By this result, it is substantiated that this docking is very effective to binding with ligands particularly with the antagonists. This also suggests that the α_7nAChR is highly sensitive to the antagonists.

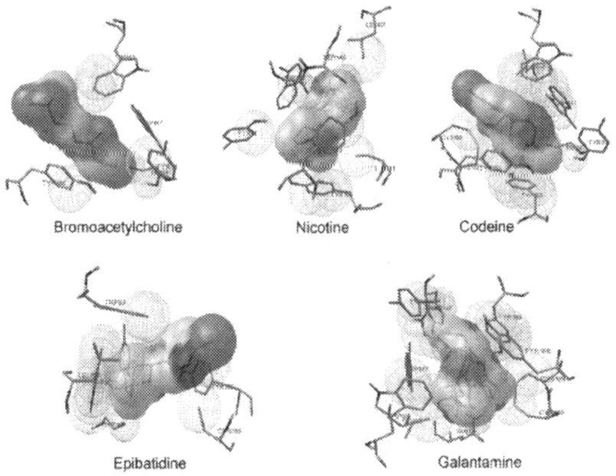

Figure 27a

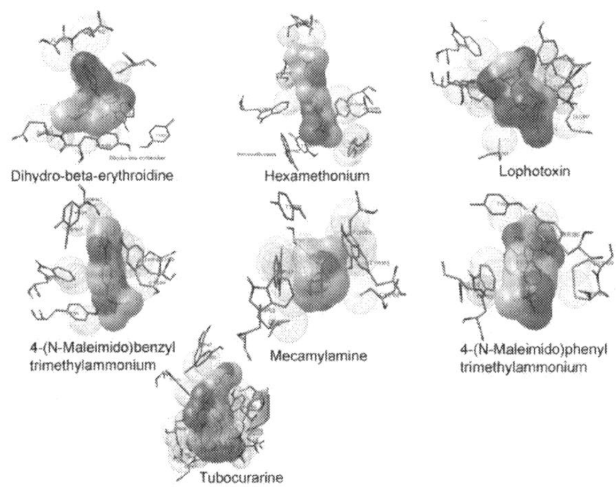

Figure 27b

Rigid ligand interaction with mutated α_7nAChR. 8A shows the agonists interacts with the mutated α_7nAChR. 8B shows the antagonists with interacts with mutated α_7nAChR. The interactions were obtained from the inbuilt module from AutoDock.

These mutation investigations can be subjected to experimental studies further, to validate and use this in effective manner in future. These results provide the details of interactions of ligands with the three dimensional model of N-terminal region of human α_7nAChR and thereby point to the design of novel lead compounds also.

Table 14: Mutation 03

S.No	Agonist	Energy Kcal/Mol	Interacting residues
1	**Bromoacetylcholine**	-6.39	LEU107,GLN115,CYS189,TYR193
2	**Nicotine**	-9.23	TRP147,SER148,TYR186,CYS189,TYR193
3	**Codeine**	-10.61	TRP53,LEU117,TRP147,TYR186,CYS188,CYS189,TYR193
4	**Epibatidine**	-10.01	TRP53,LEU117,TRP147,TYR186,CYS189
5	**Galanthamine**	-10.64	TRP53,LEU107,GLN115,LEU117,TYR146,TRP147,SER148,TYR186, CYS188,CYS189,TYR193
	Antagonist		
6	**Hexamethionium**	-6.32	TRP53,ALA161,ASP162,SER166,TYR186,CYS189,TYR193
7	**Mecalamine**	-10.06	TRP53,LEU117,TRP147,TYR186,CYS189,TYR193
8	**4-(N-**	-8.23	TRP53,TRP147,SER166,TYR186,CYS188,CYS189
9	**4-(N-**	-8.53	TRP53,LEU117,TRP147,SER148,SER166,TYR186,CYS189
10	**dihydro-beta-erythroiodine**	-8.91	ALA161,ALA162,SER166,TYR186,GLU187
11	**Lophotoxin**	-10.48	TYR34,TRP53,TYR91,ALA161,SER166,TYR186,GLU187,CYS188,C
12	**d-tubocurarine**	-10.39	TRP53,ALA161,ASP162,GLY165,SER166,ARG184,TYR186,GLU187,

The class-specific residues which were identified using docking were subjected to mutation type 3. This mutation involves the substitution of SER146 (+) with TYR, SER34 (-) with TYR, GLN55 (-) with ASN and TYR166 (-) with SER respectively using Sybyl 7.1. Mutated residues which appeared to interact with the ligand were highlighted. The results were obtained from the inbuilt module of AutoDock for analyzing the interacting residues.

Table 15: H-Bond analysis using Interactor

S.No	Ligands	Wild	M1	M2	M3
1	**Bromoacetylcholine**	GLN55	X	GLU55	X
2	**Codeine**	X	X	X	X
3	**dihydro-beta-erythroiodine**	X	X	X	X
4	**Epibatidine**	X	X	X	X
5	**Galanthamine**	X	X	X	TYR146
6	**Hexamethionine**	X	X	GLU55	X
7	**Lophotoxin**	X	X	X	SER166
8	**4-(N-Maleimido)benzyltrimethylammonium**	X	X	GLU55	X
9	**Mecalamine**	X	X	X	X
10	**4-(N-Maleimido)phenyltrimethylammonium**	X	X	GLU55	X
11	**Nicotine**	X	X	X	X
12	**d-tubocurarine**	GLN55	ALA166	GLU55	SER166

All the docked complexes were subjected to the H-bond analysis using our in-house program Interactor. The program stripped out the residues which were interacting with the respective ligand. The hydrogen bond interaction was found to occur greater in number from the mutation type 2 and 3 than from mutation type 1. This represents the mutation type 2 & 3 were of higher efficiency than from type 1. X represents no H-Bond interaction and the residue name indicates the interaction of the ligand with the corresponding residue.

Evolutionary Trace Analysis

In order to examine those impacts of mutations on the residues on conserved and class-specific regions of nAChR, a series of diverse nAChR receptors remains to be tested. However, Evolutionary Trace (ET) analysis is a sequence-structure analysis technique described by Lichtarge *et al(Lichtarge et al. 1996; Lichtarge and Sowa 2002; Ward et al. 2009)*, was applied to identify potential regions for mutagenesis in nAChR. This aims to find receptor binding specificity determinants for five major sub-groups in the family of nAChR by ET by creating an evolutionary tree using the PHYLIP package (Retief 2000). The ECD of α_2, α_3, α_4, α_7 and α_9 sequences of nAChR family were retrieved from SwissProt database and submitted to Trace Suite II server. The server produces a phylogenetic tree and a trace alignment respectively. The trace alignment produces 10 consensus sequences at each level of ETC, and the phylogenetic tree is generated from five major branches with partition ranging from P1-P10. As expected, the sequence form *Lymnaea stagnalis* stands on its own as a separate cluster and the sequence of nAChR were found to be more similar.

The trace procedure was followed automatically for each partition by TraceSeq and TraceScript which follows these steps respectively. (1) Protein sequence connected by a common node with evolutionary time greater than a given ETC value were clustered together by TraceGroup and input into TraceSeq. (2) To distinguish between conserved and non-conserved position, a consensus sequence was generated for each group. In practice, TraceSeq tagged a residue with a '1' if it was conserved or with a '0' if it varied within the subgroup. (3) By comparing the aligned consensus sequences for all the clusters associated with a given partition, a trace was generated. Where all residues for a specific position had been tagged as '1', the one-letter residue name was used if such an amino acid was found in every single cluster, otherwise the position was assigned the symbol 'X' and was termed 'Class-specific'; if an amino acid had been tagged with a '0' in at least one of the consensus sequences, the corresponding position in the trace was considered to be neutral. (4) Script files for both Rasmol (Sayle and Milner-White 1995; Goodsell 2005) and MOLSCRIPT (Esnouf 1997) were created by TraceScript to map the trace on to the surface of available structures. The various residue classes were color-coded to distinguish between conserved and class-specific, as well as buried and exposed. Residues were classified as buried if their side-chain solvent accessibility was lower than 30%.

Carrying out the analysis on five different sequence groups among the nAChR allows us to access the validity of the method. The aligned non-redundant sequences of nAChR which contains five α_2 sequences, five α_3 sequences, six α_4 sequences, six α_7 sequences, and three α_9 sequences with one AChBP sequence from *Lymnaea stagnalis* respectively. Sequences of subfamilies show high conservation among themselves, but across the subfamily there is hardly any conservation apart from the cysteines. It should be considered that Cys188-189 is also conserved among the superfamily which is said to be the identity of the superfamily. However, SER146 was absolutely conserved among all the subtypes. The polar residue SER34 is replaced by polar and aromatic residue which is present at the β_1 region, which interacts with the ligand molecules that may be important for specificity in binding. It is conserved among nicotinic type but slightly varies in the muscarnic type of nAChR. On contrast, GLN55 displays maximal sequence variation among the subtypes and TYR166 is highly conserved in nicotinic type but not in the muscarnic type, which displays minimal sequence variation, which is also confirmed by Evolutionary Trace method. However the conserved residues among the homologues sequences were found to be ~26.6%.

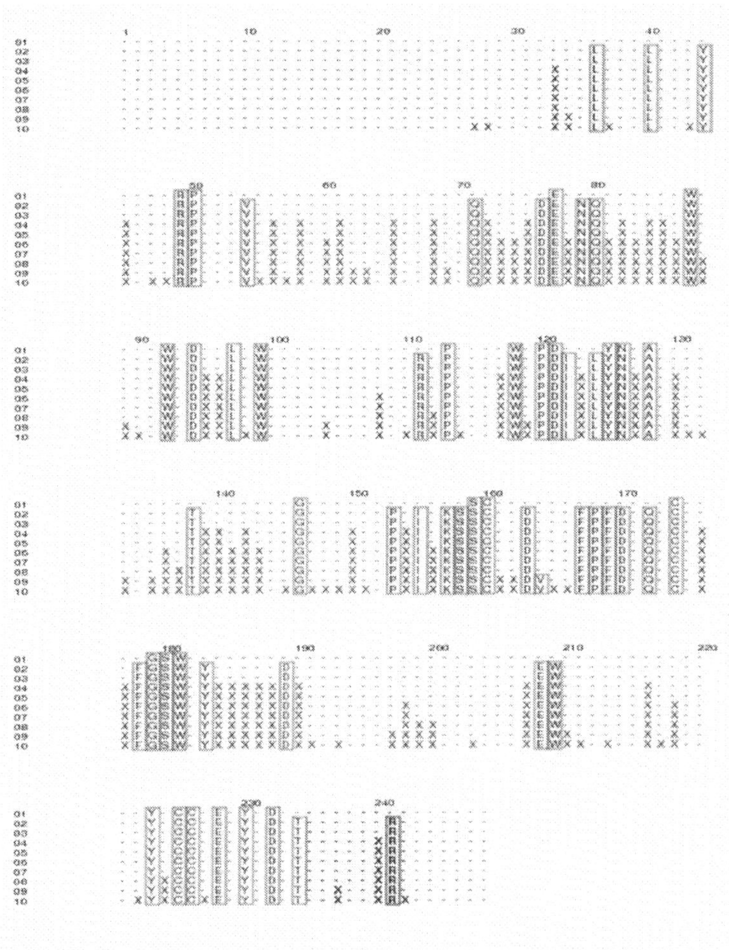

Figure 28: Evolutionary trace analysis. The extracellular domain of α_2, α_3, α_4, α_7 and α_9 of neuronal nAChR sequences were aligned for partition P1-P10. The conserved residues were displayed in yellow color; the class-specific residues were displayed in green color and the neutral residues were displayed in cyan color.

The output from the TraceSuiteII program on the ECD of nAChR is shown in [Fig. 28]. Analysis of the mapped traces for partition P1-P10 revealed clusters of potentially important residues on the binding site of the receptor. The residues defined by the hydrophobic trait are at the interface region. In the partition P01 apart from the structurally conserved cysteines at the interface region, ARG18, PRO19, GLU43, TRP53, TRP58, ASP60, LEU63, TRP65, PRO79, TRP84, PRO86, ASP87, TYR91, ASN92, ALA94, GLY112, SER125, CYS126, CYS140, GLY145, SER146, TRP147, TYR186, GLU191, TYR193 and ASP195 are absolutely conserved among the receptors of nAChR. Among the conserved residues TRP53, TYR91, TRP147, TYR186, CYS188-189 and TYR193 were found to involve at the interface region which is the binding site region. The disulphide linkage CYS126-CYS140 located between β_4 and β_7; and CYS188-CYS189 located between the loop region β_9 and β_{10} maintains the structural rigidity.

At the partition P02 LEU5, LEU9, TYR13, VAL20, GLY37, ASP42, ASN45, GLN46, LEY90, THR101, PRO119, ILE121, LYS123, SER124, ASP129, VAL130, PHE133, PRO134, PHR135, ASP136, GLN138, PHE144, TYR149, ASP155, GLY171, TRP172, TYR197 and ARG205 were found to conserve among all the α_2, α_3, α_4, α_7 and α_9 nAChR types. Among the conserved residue GLU43, TRP58, ASP60, LEU63, TRP65, PRO79, TRP84, PRO86 and ASP87 which lies away from the interface region and binding site, posses less functional importance. The residues which were present at the partition P04 were identified as class-specific region. Based on the output generated by TraceSuite the conserved, class specific and neutral residues were mapped on the surface of the theoretical model nAChR [Fig. 29] to look at their special distributions.

This ensures that the functional patches detected at the binding site of these highly related protein sequences occupy similar regions of the molecule, regardless of the functional differences. The complete sequences of these polypeptides were aligned manually, using the invariant cysteines of nAChR as anchor points. Special care was taken in ensuring the gaps were not inserted into areas of known secondary structure. A Phylip distance matrix based on sequence identity was generated from the 26 non-redundant sequences by the ClustalX program (Thompson *et al.* 2002) [Table 9] and was input into the Kitsch algorithm to build a rooted phylogenetic tree.

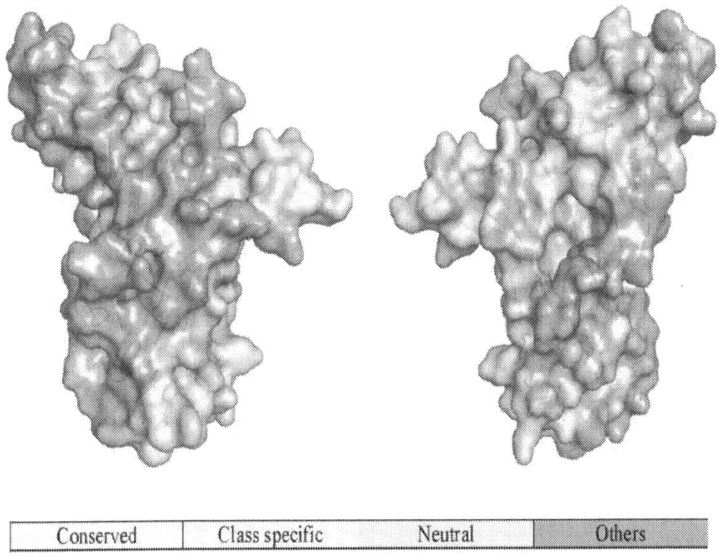

Figure 29: The evolutionary trace results were mapped over the theoretical structure of α_7nAChR. The conserved residues were segmented in yellow color; the class-specific residues were segmented in green color and the neutral residues were segmented in light cyan color.

Table 16: Table of Conserved, Class specific and Neutral residues in Extra Cellular Region of nAChR, generated based on the Trace produced by Evolutionary Trace Server.

S.No		Alpha7#		Alpha9#	Alpha2$	Alpha3$	Alpha4$
	1	5	L	L	L	L	L
		6	Y	F	F	F	L
		*7(B)	K	N	K	E	K
		8	E	D	H	R	K
	2	9	L	L	L	L	L
		10	V	F	F	F	F
		11	K	E	R	E	S
		12	N	D	G	D	G
	3	13	Y	Y	Y	Y	Y
		14	N	S	N	N	N
		*15(A)	P	N	R	E	K
		16	L	A	W	I	W
		*17(A)	E	L	A	I	S
	4	*18(A)	R	R	R	R	R
	5	*19(A)	P	P	P	P	P
	6	20	V	V	V	V	V
		21	A	P	A	A	E
		22	N	N	N	N	D
		23	D	T	V	I	T
		24	S	S	S	S	D
		25	Q	D	D	D	K
		26	P	V	P	V	V
		27	L	V	V	V	L
		28	T	I	I	L	N
		29	V	V	I	V	V
		30	Y	R	Q	R	T
		31	F	F	F	F	L
		32	S	G	E	G	Q
		33	L	L	V	L	I
		34	S	S	S	S	T
		35	L	I	M	I	L
		36	L	A	S	A	S
		*37(B)	Q	Q	Q	Q	Q
		38	I	I	L	L	L
		*39(B)	M	K	I	V	I
		40	D	D	D	K	D
		41	V	M	V	V	V
	7	42	D	D	D	D	D
	8	43	E	E	E	E	E

		44	K	R	K	V	K
	9	*45(A)	N	N	N	N	N
	10	46	Q	Q	Q	Q	Q
		47	V	I	M	I	M
		48	L	L	M	M	M
		49	T	T	T	E	T
		50	T	A	T	T	T
		51	N	Y	N	N	N
		*52(B)	I	L	V	L	V
	11	53	W	W	W	W	W
		54	L	I	L	L	V
		55	Q	R	K	K	K
		56	M	Q	Q	Q	Q
		57	S	I	E	I	E
	12	58	W	W	W	W	W
		59	T	H	S	N	H
	13	60	D	D	D	D	D
		61	H	A	Y	Y	Y
		62	Y	Y	K	K	K
	14	63	L	L	L	L	L
		64	Q	T	R	K	R
	15	65	W	W	W	W	W
	16	77	R	R	R	R	R
		78	F	I	V	V	P
	17	79	P	P	P	P	I
		80	D	S	S	A	S
		81	G	D	E	E	E
		82	Q	L	M	K	L
		83	I	V	I	I	I
	18	84	W	W	W	W	W
		*85(A)	K	R	I	K	R
	19	86	P	P	P	P	P
	20	87	D	D	D	D	D
	21	88	I	I	I	I	I
		89	L	V	V	V	V
	22	90	L	L	L	L	L
	23	91	Y	Y	Y	Y	Y
	24	*92(A)	N	N	N	N	N
		*93(A)	S	K	N	N	N
	25	*94(A)	A	A	A	A	A
		95	D	D	D	V	D
		96	E	D	G	G	G
		97	R	E	E	D	D
		*98(B)	F	S	F	F	F

		*99(B)	D	S	A	Q	A
		*100(B)	A	E	V	V	V
		101	T	P	T	D	T
		*102(B)	F	H	D	H	V
		103	H	M	K	L	N
		*104(B)	T	T	T	T	T
		105	N	K	K	K	N
		106	V	A	A	A	V
		107	L	H	L	H	V
		108	V	L	L	L	L
		109	N	F	K	F	R
		110	S	S	Y	H	Y
		111	S	T	T	D	D
		112	G	G	G	G	G
		113	H	T	E	R	L
		114	C	V	V	V	I
		115	Q	H	T	Q	T
		116	Y	W	W	W	W
		117	L	V	I	T	D
	26	119	P	P	P	P	P
		120	G	A	A	A	A
	27	121	I	I	I	I	I
		*122(A)	F	T	Y	F	Y
	28	123	K	K	K	K	K
	29	*124(A)	S	S	S	S	S
	30	125	S	S	S	S	S
	31	126	C	C	C	C	C
		127	Y	V	S	K	S
		128	I	V	I	I	I
	32	129	D	D	D	D	D
	33	130	V	V	V	V	V
		131	R	T	T	T	T
		132	W	Y	F	Y	F
	34	133	F	F	F	F	F
	35	134	P	P	P	P	P
	36	135	F	F	F	F	F
	37	136	D	D	D	D	D
		137	V	N	Q	Y	Q
	38	138	Q	Q	Q	Q	Q
		139	H	Q	N	N	N
	39	140	C	C	C	C	C
		141	K	N	K	T	T
		142	L	L	M	M	M
		*143(A)	K	T	K	K	K
	40	*144(A)	F	F	F	F	F
	41	145	G	G	G	G	G
	42	*146(A)	S	S	S	S	S

	43	*147(A)	W	W	W	W	W
		*148(A)	S	T	T	S	T
	44	*149(A)	Y	Y	Y	Y	Y
		*150(A)	G	N	D	D	D
		151	G	G	K	K	K
		152	W	N	A	A	A
		153	S	Q	K	K	K
		154	L	V	I	I	I
		155	D	D	D	D	D
		156	L	L	L	L	I
		157	Q	E	V	V	F
		158	M	Q	L	N	N
		159	Q	M	I	M	A
		160	E	E	G	H	L
		161	A	Q	S	S	D
		-	-	T	S	R	S
		-	-	V	M	V	G
		*162(B)	D	D	N	D	D
		163	I	L	L	Q	L
		164	S	K	K	L	S
		*165(B)	G	D	D	D	D
		166	Y	Y	Y	F	F
		167	I	W	W	W	I
		*168(B)	P	E	E	E	E
		169	N	S	S	S	D
		*170(B)	G	G	G	G	V
	45	171	E	E	E	E	E
	46	172	W	W	W	W	W
		173	D	A	A	V	E
		174	L	I	I	I	V
		175	V	V	I	V	H
		176	G	N	K	D	G
		177	I	A	A	A	M
		178	P	T	P	V	P
		179	G	G	G	G	A
		180	K	T	Y	T	V
		181	R	Y	K	Y	K
		182	S	N	H	N	N
		183	E	S	D	T	V
		184	R	K	I	R	I
	47	185	Y	Y	Y	Y	Y
		*186(A)	E	G	D	N	E
	48	*187(A)	C	C	C	C	C

	49	*188(A)	C	C	C	C	C
		189	K	S	A	E	A
	50	190	E	E	E	E	E
		191	P	P	I	I	I
	51	192	Y	Y	Y	Y	Y
	52	193	P	P	P	P	P
	53	194	D	D	D	D	D
		195	V	V	V	I	I
	54	196	T	T	T	T	T
		197	F	F	Y	Y	Y
		198	T	T	A	S	A
		199	V	L	F	L	F
		200	T	L	V	Y	V
		201	M	L	I	I	I
		202	R	K	R	R	R
		203	R	R	R	R	R

The conserved, class-specific residues were highlighted using yellow and green color. Among the group of nAChR subunit type # forms Homopentamer, $ forms Heteropentamer and the * forms Residues at the Interface region. The conserved residue among the homologues sequence **~ 26.6 %.**

Phylogenetic tree

The partitions ranges from P01 to P10 divide the phylogenetic tree into respective groups based on appropriate classes. An individual partition contains different numbers of classes, where each class consists of a cluster of similar sequences originating from a common node within the respective partition [Fig. 30]. From the root, nodes 1 and 2 were originated at the level of partition P01. One of these branches contains the AChBP sequence, while the other branch consists of the remaining nAChR sequences, indicating that the AChBP sequences may indeed constitute an independent and distinct to nAChR. The partition P03 discriminates into node3 in which α_9 group is collated into a single branch and node4 which comprises rest of α groups. However, the partition P04 further divides into node5 and node6, in which α_7 sequences were grouped into single branch and rest of the α_2, α_3, α_4 groups into partition P06. At the partition P06, node 7 & 8 were further classified into α_3 group and α_2, α_4 groups respectively. The partition P08 grouped into two different clusters of α_2, α_4 groups at 9th and 10th node, which lies proximal to each other respectively.

Thus, the ET method can be used both to rationalize the result of the mutagenesis studies and to predict the novel leads for neurodegenerative diseases.

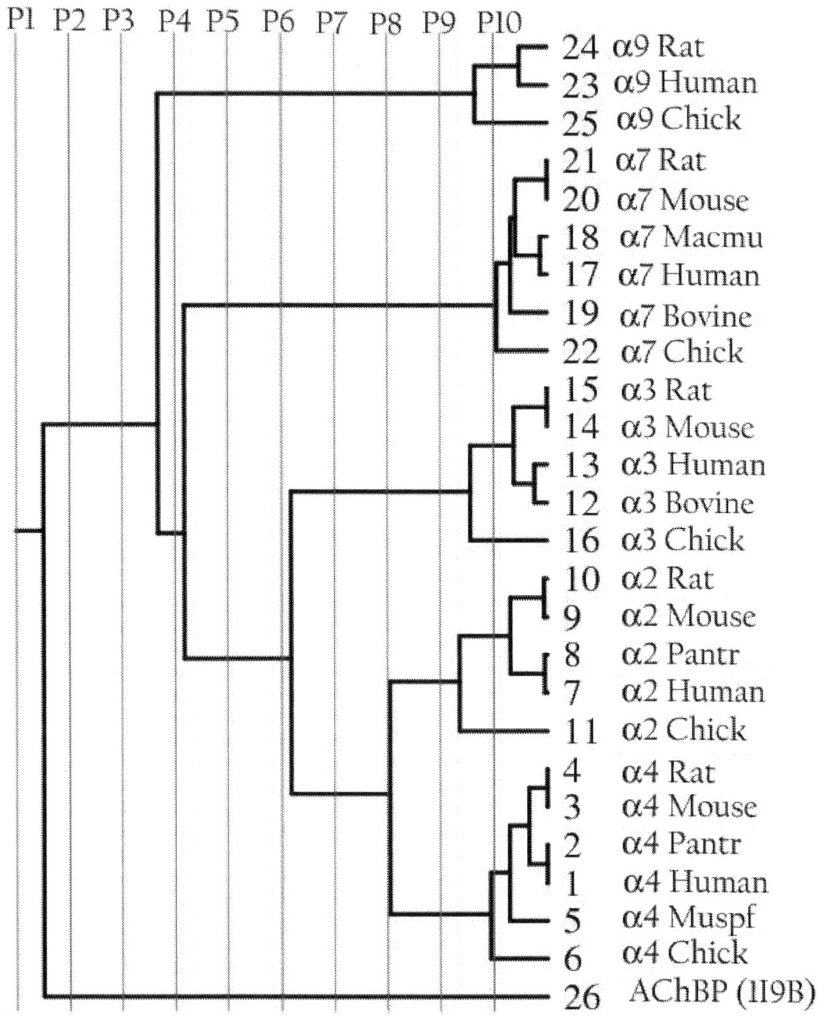

Figure 30: Dendrogram containing 26 sequences of ECD of nAChR family, selected using Phylip 3.5 on the basis of sequence dissimilarity.

4. Molecular Dynamics Studies of Human Neuronal α_7nAChR with Agonist and Antagonists.

Homology Modelling of α_7nAChR

In our previous studies, using homology modeling approach, a theoretical model of α_7nAChR was constructed based on the homologous structure AChBP from great pond snail as the structural template solved at 2.7Å using Modeller9v2 (Sali and Blundell 1993). One representative structure was selected from the Modeller run, based on minimum energy. The protomer thus generated was assembled into pentamer based on the initial equivalencies from EBI-Dalilite server using InsightII and subsequently minimized using Sybyl7.1 up to 100 iterations to remove the steric clashes at the interfaces. Molecular docking studies was performed with a cluster of small molecule which is agonists and antagonists in its nature (Parthiban *et al.* 2009).

Molecular Docking with agonists and antagonists

Based on the brief literature survey (Arias 1997; Arias 2000), our earlier study was extended on molecluar interaction on array of agonists and antagonists which targets α_7nAChR. These ligand molecules were selected from PubChem database. The molecules were then subjected to VLifeMDS suite for optimizing the molecules for steric clashes and geometric inaccuracies. The nAChR were then targeted by all these agonists and antagonists focusing particularly at the interface region. The dockings of these agonists and the antagonists were carried out in two different approaches. (i) The ligands were allowed to rotate freely during the docking and hence it is flexible ligand docking. (ii) The ligands were not allowed to rotate by reducing its torsion angles, with the aim of forming same interaction between ligand and receptor. Hence it is rigid ligand docking. The docking results were analyzed further and the interactions were examined visually using analyzing interaction module present in AutoDock and tabulated. It was observed that the interacting residues were mostly common to both the docking types. But it was noted that the binding energy was remarkably much higher for rigid ligand interaction than flexible interaction. With this information the agonists and antatonists which interact with the receptor with best binding energy were selected as a representative for docking and preceded with the molecular dynamics studies. Since, nAChR is highly sensitive to toxins; we preferred to select

Lophotoxin, a marine neurotoxin which covalently react with nAChR (Groebe and Abramson 1995) for this current study.

Molecular Dynamics simulation of α_7nAChR with explicit solvent model

To our knowledge, this is the first time that the theoretical model of ECD of human neuronal α_7nAChR in open state have been generated and equilibrated in solution mixture in apo state and bound with agonist and antagonists using MD simulations. In this, nAChR bound to agonist and antagonists interaction were studied in terms of (1) nature of stability maintained by active-site residues, interacting with the ligands throughout the simulation, (2) interaction of the solvent with the ligand molecule (3) monitoring the C-loop fluctuation in terms of its movement in due course towards or away from the interacting ligand.

Structural stability and Dynamics

The theoretical pentameric model of ECD of human neuronal α_7nAChR in open channel state was maintained reasonably well, and the pentameric structure was reduced to dimer for consistency as well, and is believed that this result is applicable to all the subunits. It is considered that the binding of ligand at single interface region is identical for all the subunits. Figure shows the top and side views structure of the α_7nAChR after 10ns of MD simulations. All the simulations were tested for stability by examining energies, root-mean square deviation (RMSD) and root-mean square fluctuation (RMSF) and radius of gyration (R_g).

Mean square deviation

The overall stability of the model was evaluated using the root-mean square deviation (RMSD) [Fig. 31] of backbone atoms away from their initial homology model positions. The RMSD is an indicator of the structural stability of a protein in a given environment.

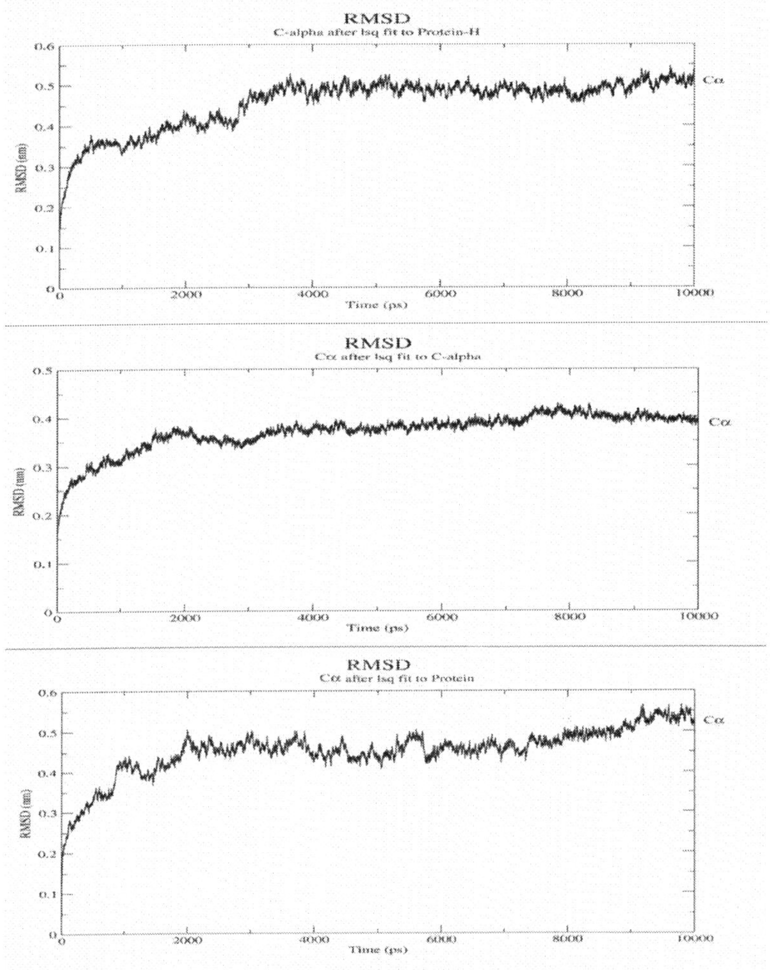

Figure 31. RMSD of the theoretical model nAChR calculated against initial structure for apo state and ligand bound state for 10ns simulation. (a). Apo state (B). Theoretical model of nAChR bound to agonist galanthamine and (C) theoretical model of nAChR bound to lophotoxin.

The theoretical model of α_7nAChR in apo increases rapidly at first, owing to thermal vibrations and improper interaction. Later it was found to stabilize initially till 3ns consistently and finally reaches a stable conformation to get stabilized equilibrium position after 3ns. Rest of the simulation suggests a balanced system indicating that the homology model provides a reasonable starting structure for the simulations. The α_7nAChR bound to agonist galanthamine were stabilized well after 2ns after an immediate raise during the initial period of the dynamics. Simultaneously, the α_7nAChR bound to antagonist lophotoxin gets stabilized well after 2ns vigorously after an initial raise during the initial period of the dynamics. After 7ns the equilibrium position increases slightly and is maintained. After 9ns it takes an additional equilibrium position, unable to maintain its pervious equilibrium state. Based on this stabilization it is clear that nAChR is more sensitive and unstable to antagonists than agonist interactions by means of structural maintenance mainly at loop regions. Moreover, this additional equilibrium state can shift to another equilibrium or it can come back to retain its native state. This can be performed when the simulation can be extended more than 10ns [36]. In the absence of ligand, the binding site residues were found more collapsed than when ligand is bound state, and this was well quantified by following up the distance Cys189-189 during the simulation period.

Mean square fluctuation.

An extensive flexibility of the models was characterized by estimating the root-mean square fluctuation (RMSF) of the Cα atoms over the 10ns simulations. A RMSF provides more detailed information on the mobility of the residues relative to the average structure. The RMSF of apo state, agonist and antagonists formed as a complex of the LBD are shown in [Fig. 32]. This approach calculates the average fluctuation in a given window and can be used as an indicator of sampling a given conformational state [37]. The simulations of nAChR in the apo state displays elevated movement in the RMSF plots than the nAChR bound with galanthamine and lophotoxin. Perhaps, indicating a degree of structural stability resulting from the presence of the ligand.

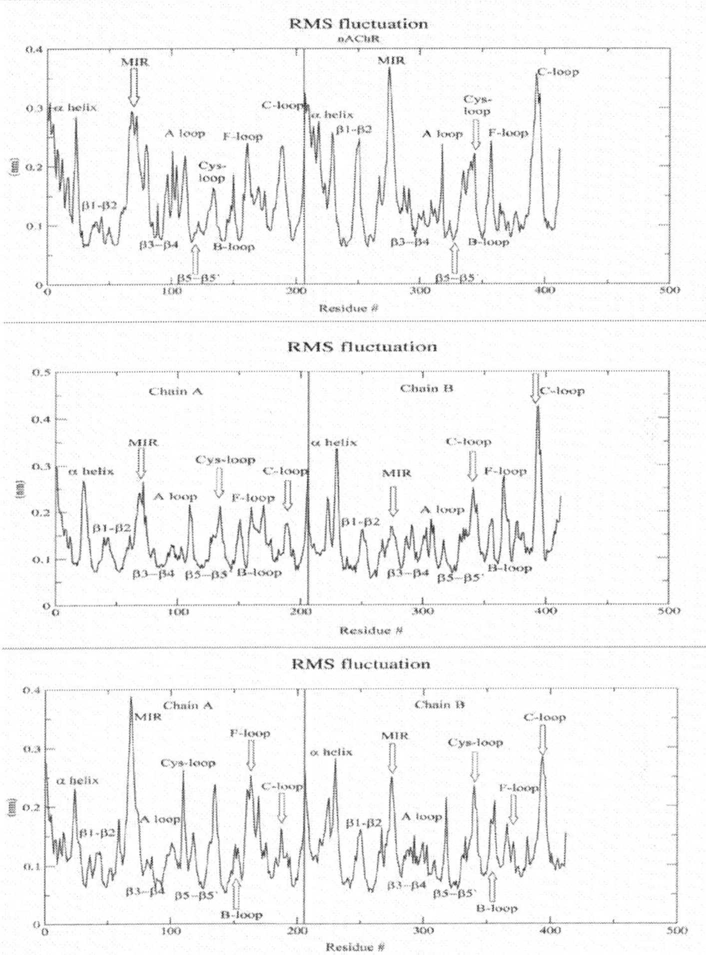

Figure 32. RMSF of the theoretical model nAChR calculated against initial C□ for apo state and ligand bound state for 10ns simulation. (a). Theoretical model of nAChR in Apo state (B). Theoretical model of nAChR bound to agonist galanthamine and (C) theoretical model of nAChR bound to lophotoxin.

For nAChR-ligand complex, these fluctuations become more intense in fluctuation at the C-loop region present at the interface region. It seems that the increase in fluctuations in C-loop regions is concerted. There is an explanation for this intense fluctuation in C-loop, because these are the regions directly involved in interaction with a bulky ligands/toxin molecule, therefore the motions of residues there are more restricted.

Several loops, including MIR and C-loop which is crucial for ligand binding showed significantly higher flexibility at the interface region. However, in all simulations, the RMSF values continue to show higher flexibility in many loop regions and minimal variation in secondary structure region which indicates that the conformational dynamics of the protein as a whole are far from being fully sampled.

Radius of Gyration

The radius of gyration R_g is a measure of compactness of EC domain of nAChR [Fig 33] and is used as a pointer for protein stability during the simulation [38]. The R_g was applied to ligand free and ligand bound to receptor throughout the length of the simulation. The R_g of receptor interacting with agonist takes the equilibrium position from 6^{th}ns onwards and maintain thereafter. Simultaneously, the receptor interacting with lophotoxin takes an equilibrium place from 1ns onwards. Later from 7ns onwards equilibrium position devaluates slightly to take additional equilibrium position from 9ns onwards and continues after 10ns. This type of change in equilibrium happened in RMSD of lophotoxin also. This indicates that when lophotoxin or other antagonists interacts with nAChR the receptor was highly sensitive, also when the receptor was free from ligand the R_g landscape indicates the instability in maintaining the equilibrium state.

Energy

The simulated system with nAChRs were sampled with the potential, kinetic and total energy components [Fig. 34] were found to be constant across the simulation, which is typical of a temperature-coupled system at 300K.

DSSP

The DSSP algorithm is the standard method for assigning secondary structure of the amino acids of the protein given the atomic-resolution coordinates of the protein. This algorithm is applied for receptor of apo state and bound to its agonist galanthamine and antagonists Lophotoxin, which gives out a strip graph [Fig 35]. This displays that secondary structure of the dimer was maintaining its stability through the simulation period indicating that secondary structure have not got altered drastically throughout the simulation.

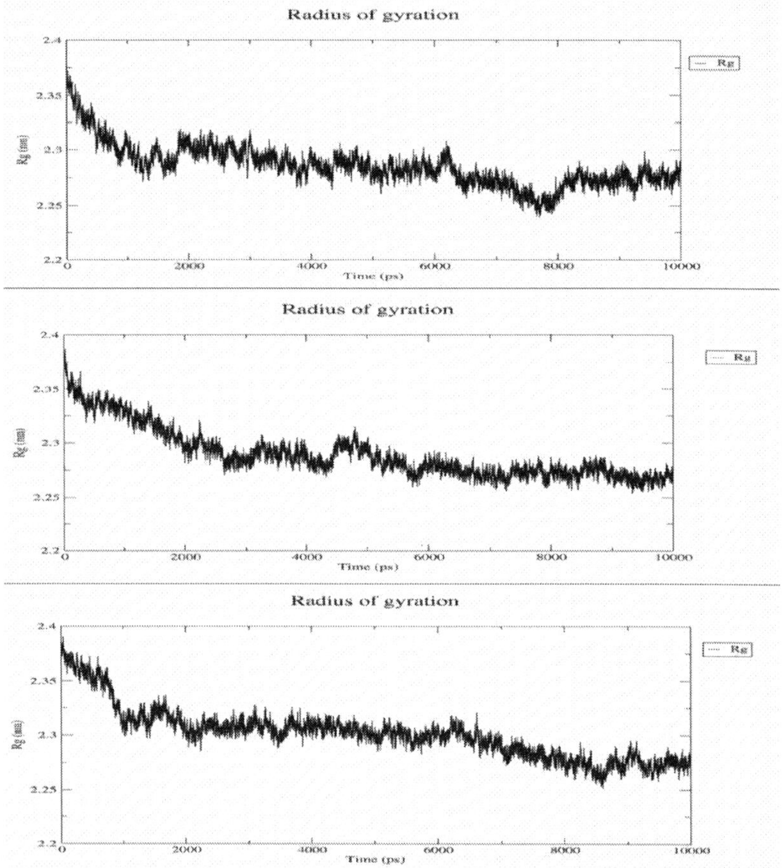

Figure 33. R_g of the theoretical model nAChR calculated against initial structure for apo state and ligand bound state for 10ns simulation. (a). Theoretical model of nAChR in Apo state (B). Theoretical model of nAChR bound to agonist galanthamine and (C) theoretical model of nAChR bound to lophotoxin.

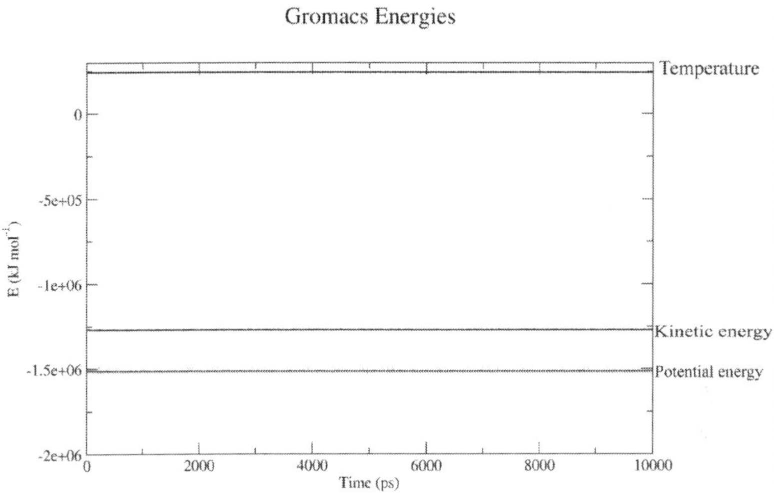

Figure 34. The energies were calculated for the theoretical model of nAChR after 10ns simulation. The black color indicates the temperature; blue color indicates the kinetic energy and the red color indicates the potential energy. All these energies were maintained during the molecular dynamics simulation.

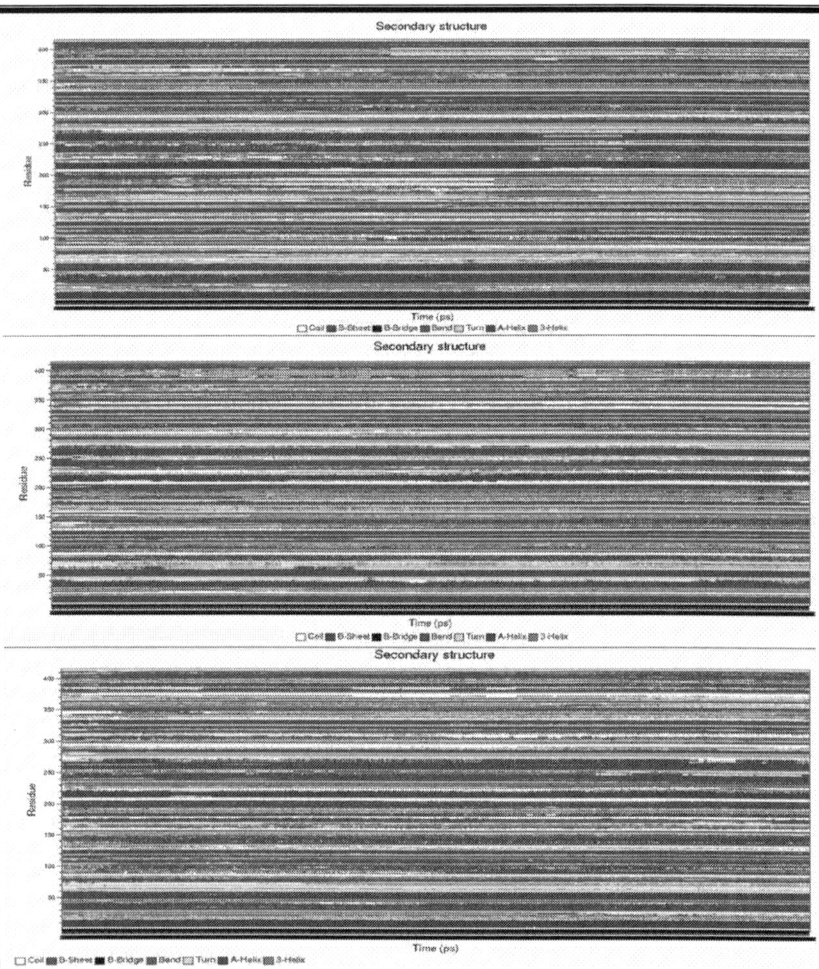

Figure 35: DSSP was calculated for the theoretical model of nAChR after 10ns simulation. (a). theoretical structure in Apo state (B) theoretical structure of nAChR with galanthamine (C) theoretical structure of nAChR with Lophotoxin. The strip graph indicates the structural stability was maintained in the secondary structure.

These indicate that, as expected, the MD protocol is well suited to assessing the stability of the theoretical model of α_7nAChR.

Analyzing Ligand Flexibility at binding-site region

The flexibility of the ligands within the binding site was examined further. The ligands for both the galanthamine and lophotoxin simulations maintained their position well within the binding pocket for the duration of the simulation. Although both ligands held their place and general orientations in the binding pocket, galanthamine was much more rigid than lophotoxin in terms of availability rotatable bonds. Analysis of the rotatable bonds has shown a fairly rigid conformation of galanthamine, consistent with few binding mode that differs only by a slight tilting of the ring at the core structure. The rotatable angle for lophotoxin shows more flexibility of the chain when compared with galanthamine. The molecule maintains its orientation well, but there are rotations at all the sides of the ligands outer side suggesting multiple conformations may be equally favorable within the pocket. Docking studies also suggest that galanthamine has less mode of binding while lophotoxin may have more than that of galanthamine.

Movement of C-Loop at the interface region

It would be expected that different structural changes take place in binding sites and at the subunit interfaces. It is suggested that the two alpha subunits have an "open" arrangement in the "resting" of nAChR (Brejc *et al.* 2001), making the ligand-binding pocket accessible to the agonist/antagonist binding. An important motion in the simulation takes place in the C-loop region [Fig 36] that forms one side of the binding site (main side). This analysis was performed visually using PyMol but superimposing the model obtained from every nanosecond after the simulations.

An interesting observation in the binding site is the "flapping" of the C-loop in the interface region in the apo forms. This confirms that the C-loop is not stable in apo conformations and does actually a continuous swing in and outward very minor range. In the case of nAChR-galanthamine complex the loop keeps moves constantly inside towards ligand. After an initial movement of the loop towards ligand till 4ns a drastic

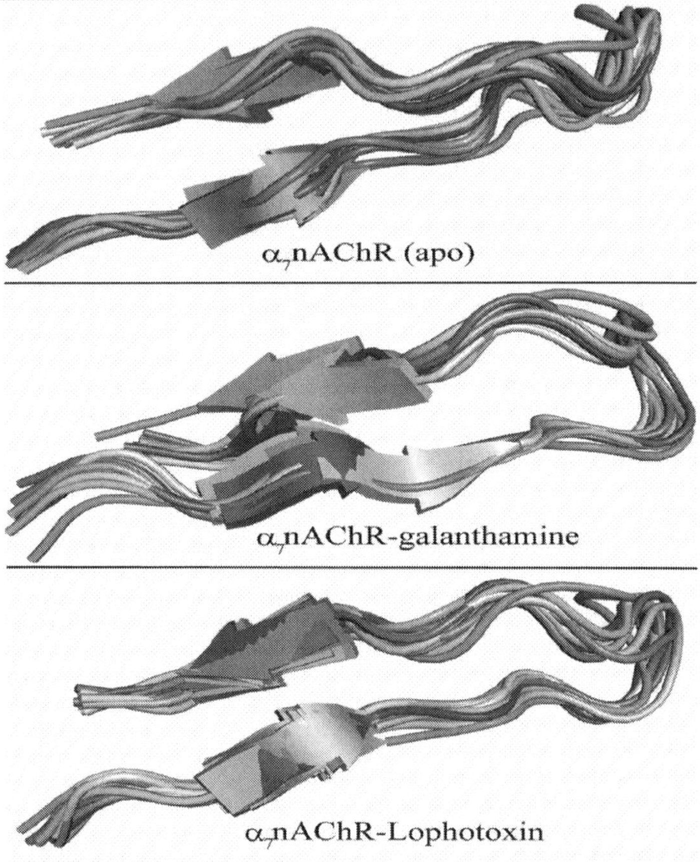

Figure 36: The C-loop movements obtained from every time ranging from 0-10ns time frame after MD. The structures were superposed using Pymol and examined visually. The dark green indicates the initial structure; rest of the colors indicates the C-loop movement during the MD simulation. (a). The C-loop highly fluctuates in the apo state. (b). The C-loop approaches towards the ligand galanthamine. (C). The C-loop swings out from the ligand Lophotoxin.

changes was observed. Subsequently, the loop constantly takes the same position and keeps flapping over there itself to hold the ligand firmly. This presence of ligand in the binding pocket makes the loop to move towards inside. On the other-side in nAChR-lophotoxin complex, the loop constantly moves outside form the receptor by holding the massive toxin molecule very firmly. After an initial stabilization from 0ns the loop flaps only up to 2ns, thereafter till 5ns the loop holds the same position. From 6^{th}ns, further changes in position outwards very slowly for rest of the simulation for every 1ns was observed. The C-loop movement is apparently limited at the interface region, owing to the presence of the bulky toxin molecules in the binding site; the interactions with binding site and C-loop therefore restrict movements in this region. The situation is almost same when RMSD was taken into consideration. The time at which the receptor stabilizes was almost the same with that of mean square deviation data.

Protein-ligand Interaction.

The protein-ligand interactions were examined by extracting different frames from the trajectory for agonist and antagonist. The frames ranging from initial of 0^{th}ns till 10^{th}ns of the simulation respectively.

All these frames were then subjected to Ligplot server [Fig. 33] to examine the crucial residues interacting with the ligand molecule. The receptor maintains interaction with Tyr91, Trp147, Tyr186, Cys188-189, Tyr193, Trp259, Gln261, Leu313, Gln321 and Leu323 with galanthamine. The residues like Tyr186, Cys188 and Tyr193 forms hydrogen bond, but failed to maintain its stability further. Tyr149 which newly interacts with ligand and forms a hydrogen bond was maintained till the end of simulation. Trp259, Gln261, Tyr149 and Gln321 were found to interact only after 1ns. Later those residues also involved in maintaining the stability of the ligand binding at the interface region. On the other-side, the receptor makes a stable interaction with Tyr186, Cys188-189, Tyr193, Ser238, Leu239, Ser240, Gln261, Asp368, Ser370 and Tyr372 throughout the simulation with Lophotoxin. Among this Tyr193 and Ser240 which maintains a strong Hydrogen bond after 1^{st}ns of the simulation. But, Ser238, Asp368 and Ser370 were also involved in hydrogen bonding; however, the bond formation was not found to be stable throughout the simulation. Some new interacting residues like Leu241, Gln321, Leu323 and Gln363 were also found; but failed to maintain its interaction in entire simulation.

Similarly, the frames collected at different time were subjected to the in-house program INTERACTOR. The program lists out possible strong interactions such as hydrogen bonds directly and those that are not mediated by water and also lists out residues that interact closely with the ligand. The analysis was performed for the entire frame, sampled at every single ns of simulation till the 10ns run of nAChR. Most of the residue which interacts with ligand coincides with Ligplot results (data not shown) in the case of both agonist and antagonist. The Hydrogen bond was formed between the receptor and ligand molecule in between the simulation and have destroyed as well.

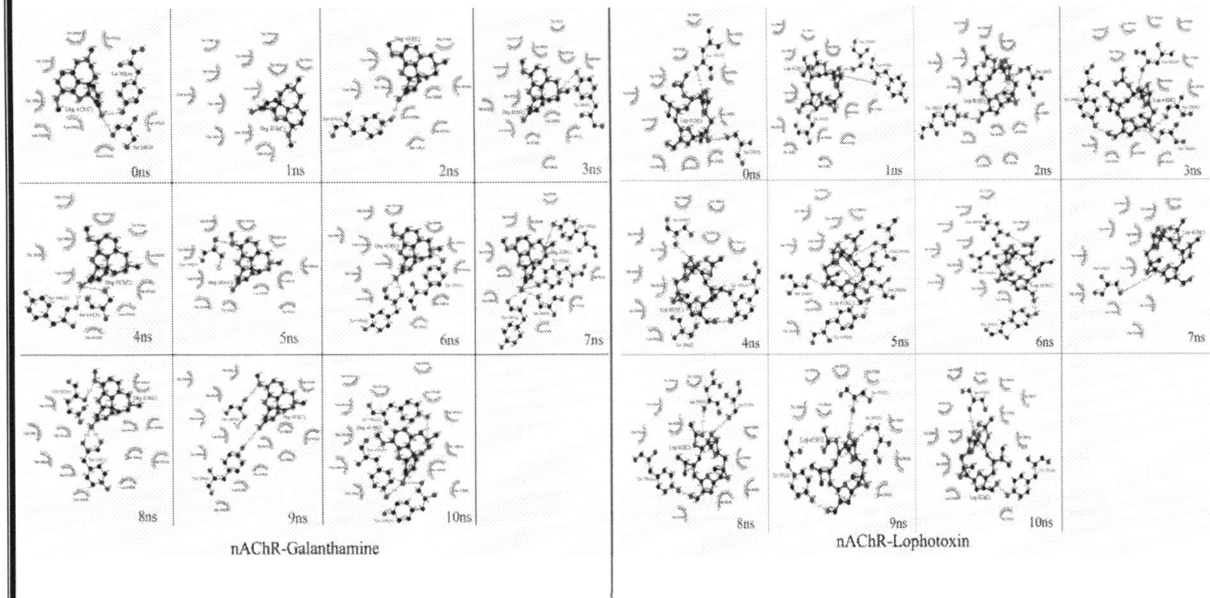

Figure 33: The protein-ligand interaction was obtained from every time frame ranging from 0-10ns time frame after MD. The interactions of theoretical model with agonists galanthamine and antagonists lophotoxin was examined using Ligplot. The presence of Hydrogen bond was indicated using dotted lines.

Water Mediated Interaction.

This interaction confirms that the importance of water molecule and its active role in protein interfaces. This also suggests that consideration of solvent in the development of energetic functions in protein interactions is essential. Moreover, the introduction of water-mediated interactions into protein interface should be substantially increasing the accuracy of protein interaction predictions. The protein-ligand coordinates which obtained from simulation was subjected to in-house program STRIPWATER. The program strips out the water molecule near the residue of desire. It has been observed that many water molecules were present at the interface region. These water molecules which were present at these interface region play a vital role in maintaining the structural stability by forming hydrogen bond directly with the ligand or mediated through water.

We believe that the results obtained from this work could be useful for deeper understanding of the physico-chemical properties underlying protein-ligand interactions in order to improve the accuracy of protein folding, docking and rational drug design methods. To our knowledge this is the first attempt to work on α_7nAChR to investigate the stability of binding site with the help of agonist and antagonist molecule.

Insilico modeling and molecular dynamics studies were carried earlier. In this docking of long chain α-neurotoxin to the theoretical model was also carried out. The major goal was to observe and compare the conformational changes in the LBD in the presence of these antagonists over a period of time, and to examine the structural determinants that govern the binding of two potent antagonists of different sizes (Nasiripourdori *et al.* 2009).

The Insilico model on α4β2 was constructed for TM domain and molecular dynamics studies carried on this. Many insight studies related to channel gating were revealed in this study. In this the Non-synchronized TM2 helices could lead to changes in side-chain orientations of pore-lining residues. They elucidated that reorientation of one or two hydrophobic side chains was enough for channel opening (Haddadian *et al.* 2008).

Another study on nAChR TM domain is to mimic the pulsive action on ACh binding, non equilibrium MD simulations were performed using Streed Rotation Molecular Dynamics method developed. The result confirmed all the motions derived from the Conventional Molecular Dynamics simulation and Normal Mode Analysis. The SRMD simulation indicated that the channel may undergo an open to close motion (Liu *et al.* 2008).

Conclusion

Insight Modeling and Docking studies

The structural information about the theoretical model of α_7 Nicotinic Acetylcholine Receptor would be valuable in the novel lead discovery for neurodegenerative diseases. These receptors have gained increased attention, since they modulate the neurotransmission at pre and post synaptic gorge. Since its hydrophobic character hampers the experimental structure yet to be solved, we have made an attempt to model the theoretical structure of N-terminal region of Ligand Binding Domain of human α_7nAChR. The model was found to be satisfactory as assessed by various servers. The ligand binding site is globally conserved and is crucial for pharmacological activity. The theoretical model was docked with peptide (α-Bungarotoxin) and non peptide (Acetylcholine, Nicotine) molecules. The ligands target the interface region of the theoretical pentamer and are buried in aromatic and hydrophobic clusters. The predicted residues involved in binding site are well conserved when compared with AChBP and potentially produces hydrophobic types of interactions with the ligand. These studies provide an insight into the nature of agonist and competitive antagonist binding with the theoretical model of α_7nAChR which will provide improved understanding towards designing the novel lead compounds. The predicted model of ligand binding domain of nAChR and the docking studies can point to experimental and mutational investigations.

Point Mutation and Evolutionary Trace analysis

The interaction studies of various ligands on the theoretical model of nAChR would be of more valuable in the lead discovery. These receptors have gained increased attention among the ion channels, since they modulate the neurotransmission at pre and post synaptic gorge. The theoretical model of α_7nAChR was generated in our previous study which was later subjected to receptor-ligand docking studies.

The ligands correspond to agonist and antagonists function was retrieved from the PubChem databases in the form of 2D representation. The ligands were processed in such a way that it can be used ready for docking with the theoretical α_7nAChR. The grid is reasonably placed at the ligand binding site, i.e., at interface region which is located between the subunits, is globally conserved and is crucial for pharmacological activity. These ligands were buried in the aromatic and hydrophobic clusters located at the interface region. The further analysis reveals that SER146, SER34, GLN55 and TYR166 were identified novel, which lie on the interface region may expect to play an additional important role in the ligand binding specificity.

These newly formed residues were subjected to Insilico point mutagenesis and further extended to docking studies to examine the occurrences of these residues is not a random occurrences for interacting the receptor. Insilico point mutagenesis experiments were therefore designed in such a way to permit us for a clear investigation made between (i) contributions to the residues at the interface region (ii) stability of the ligand binding and (iii) contributions to its ability to interact with other proteins. The mutations were of three types, which revealed the mutated class-specific residues interacting with the agonists and the antagonists. Subsequently the H-bond analysis was performed using our inhouse program Interactor to examine the occurrences of bonded interaction. The result reveals some interaction of class-specific mutated residues with the receptor.

As a support to the docking studies, the Evolutionary Trace analyses were also performed on the homologues sequences of neuronal nAChRs. The ET results listed out the potential residues as the most conserved and class-specific one, which might be important for the receptor's interaction with agonists and antagonists. Moreover the ET analysis was found to be consistent with the above mentioned docking studies on the receptor, suggesting similar residues are the crucial one for its interaction. These residues present at one of the loop region at the β_1, β_2 and β_7 regions which may be interacting with the ligands very effectively, and is also identified by ET analysis, which shows good agreement with docking results.

The role played by all conserved residues and the class-specific residues highlighted in our analysis should be further investigated by experimental mutagenesis studies. Detailed studies of the five major α subunits of nicotinic nAChR subgroups enabled us to understand the role of residues involved in the interaction in the formation of nAChR-ligand complexes. Hence it may be helpful to us in the designing of therapeutic leads agents for neurodegenerative diseases respectively.

Molecular Dynamics

Our earlier studies focus on two different aspects, one is to model the three dimensional structure of α_7nAChR and another is to perform molecular docking with an array of ligands targeting to this model to explore about conserved and class-specific residues. The quality of *in-silico* models, or how well the models reflect "true" structures, is always in question until the "true" structures become available. However, multiple evaluations on the structures indicated that model reflect previously reported characteristics of the α_7nAChR pretty well. The model developed herein should prove useful for many potential applications, such as predicting drug targets and understanding channel gating mechanism.

In our current work, MD simulations is applied to study the theoretical model of α_7nAChR to reveal the basic features of the structure and dynamics of this protein. In addition the theoretical structure has been related to more general features towards interaction of an agonist galanthamine and an antagonists lophotoxin respectively. It is focused in three different aspects; (i) stability of the receptor molecule when protein-ligand interacts, (ii) protein-solvent interaction and (iii) C-loop movement although the course of entire simulation. The result revealed by several output from Gromacs inbuilt options.

Initially, the structural stability was analyzed using RMSD, RMSF, R_g, and DSSP. All these results revealed that the receptor in the apo form is highly unstable. But when the receptor is accessible to ligands, the RMSF result revealed that the receptor undergoes higher fluctuation, particularly at the loop region. The movement of C-loop was also examined and its result revealed the same. This explains how the C-loop which acts as principle component for ligand interaction and present at the interface region, approaches or swings out from the ligand during the simulation time. The secondary structure was maintained very well throughout the simulation; this was obtained using the DSSP result in both apo and complexed state.

Subsequently, the protein-ligand interaction was analyzed using Ligplot and our in-house program Interactor. The protein-ligand complexes were obtained from the different time frame of the simulation and the analysis was performed over these complexes. The ligand is likely to interact with the residues at the interface region. The residues like Tyr91, Trp147, Tyr186,

Cys188-189, Tyr193, Trp259, Gln261, Leu313, Gln321 and Leu323 which is found to interact with the galanthamine in common throughout the simulation. The residues like Tyr186, Cys188 and Tyr193 forms hydrogen bond but is not stable throughout the simulation. But, Tyr149 which is an unexpected component forms a hydrogen bond stable till the end of simulation. On the other side when examining the antagonists Tyr186, Cys188-189, Tyr193, Ser238, Leu239, Ser240, Gln261, Asp368, Ser370 and Tyr372 makes interaction with Lophotoxin. Among these residues Tyr193 and Ser240 forms stable hydrogen bond throughout the simulation. The results revealed from the in-house program Interactor coincides with the Ligplot results.

The water-mediated interaction is analyzed using another in-house program STRIPWATER. The program strips out the neighboring water from residues of our interest. The active site residues were focused for this analysis obtained through different time frame of the simulation. These water molecules are aimed to play a vital role in maintaining the structural stability by forming hydrogen bond with either receptor or with ligand molecule.

The model derived from our earlier study has shown to accord with experimental structure AChBP, proving the validity of our model. Further, our docking study confirm the claim that nAChR is in open conformational state that favor binding of ligand to galanthamine and to lophotoxin in nature. The overall result confirms that LBD of α_7nAChR behaves in a dynamic nature in both apo state and also when complexed with ligand. Each subunit behaves specifically and individually, which results in the formation of homo-pentamer conformation of the receptor. This suggests an intensive role in the binding-to-gating mechanism. It should be mentioned that this displacement is not the only allosteric link between binding and gating, but it can give clue on how the cascade of interactions is triggered at the early stages of binging.

The comprehensive in-depth studies of these structures guides towards the advances in drug discovery/design focusing on new selective nAChR compounds. These new compounds which are designed may be agonists or antagonists in activity that selectively target the receptor and could maximize the desired effect and should minimize the side-effect. Toxins bind with higher affinity than endogenous ligands; therefore an accurate prediction of their binding mode will enable the designing of more efficient lead compounds. Further studies are required to understand the role of the dynamics in the biological function of α_7nAChR.

References

Adams, D. J., *et al.* (2003). "Omega-conotoxin CVID inhibits a pharmacologically distinct voltage-sensitive calcium channel associated with transmitter release from preganglionic nerve terminals." J Biol Chem **278**(6): 4057-62.

Altschul, S. F., *et al.* (1990). "Basic local alignment search tool." J Mol Biol **215**(3): 403-10.

Altschul, S. F. and D. J. Lipman (1990). "Protein database searches for multiple alignments." Proc Natl Acad Sci U S A **87**(14): 5509-13.

Apweiler, R., *et al.* (1997). "Protein sequence annotation in the genome era: the annotation concept of SWISS-PROT+TREMBL." Proc Int Conf Intell Syst Mol Biol **5**: 33-43.

Arias, H. R. (1997). "Topology of ligand binding sites on the nicotinic acetylcholine receptor." Brain Res Brain Res Rev **25**(2): 133-91.

Arias, H. R. (1998). "Binding sites for exogenous and endogenous non-competitive inhibitors of the nicotinic acetylcholine receptor." Biochim Biophys Acta **1376**(2): 173-220.

Arias, H. R. (1998). "Noncompetitive inhibition of nicotinic acetylcholine receptors by endogenous molecules." J Neurosci Res **52**(4): 369-79.

Arias, H. R. (2000). "Localization of agonist and competitive antagonist binding sites on nicotinic acetylcholine receptors." Neurochem Int **36**(7): 595-645.

Arias, H. R. and M. P. Blanton (2000). "Alpha-conotoxins." Int J Biochem Cell Biol **32**(10): 1017-28.

Arias, H. R., *et al.* (2001). "Interaction of barbiturate analogs with the Torpedo californica nicotinic acetylcholine receptor ion channel." Mol Pharmacol **60**(3): 497-506.

Armishaw, C., *et al.* (2009). "Rational design of alpha-conotoxin analogues targeting alpha7 nicotinic acetylcholine receptors: improved antagonistic activity by incorporation of proline derivatives." J Biol Chem **284**(14): 9498-512.

Armishaw, C. J. and P. F. Alewood (2005). "Conotoxins as research tools and drug leads." Curr Protein Pept Sci **6**(3): 221-40.

Armishaw, C. J., *et al.* (2006). "Alpha-selenoconotoxins, a new class of potent alpha7 neuronal nicotinic receptor antagonists." J Biol Chem **281**(20): 14136-43.

Bairoch, A. and R. Apweiler (1997). "The SWISS-PROT protein sequence data bank and its supplement TrEMBL." Nucleic Acids Res **25**(1): 31-6.

Bairoch, A. and R. Apweiler (1997). "The SWISS-PROT protein sequence database: its relevance to human molecular medical research." J Mol Med **75**(5): 312-6.

Barrantes, F. J. (1997). "The acetylcholine receptor ligand-gated channel as a molecular target of disease and therapeutic agents." Neurochem Res **22**(4): 391-400.

Barrantes, F. J., *et al.* (2000). "The neuronal nicotinic acetylcholine receptor in some hereditary epilepsies." Neurochem Res **25**(5): 583-90.

Benie, A. J., *et al.* (2000). "Solution structure of alpha-conotoxin SI." FEBS Lett **476**(3): 287-95.

Berman, H. M., *et al.* (2000). "The Protein Data Bank and the challenge of structural genomics." Nat Struct Biol **7 Suppl**: 957-9.

Berman, H. M., *et al.* (2000). "The Protein Data Bank." Nucleic Acids Res **28**(1): 235-42.

Bourne, Y., *et al.* (2005). "Crystal structure of a Cbtx-AChBP complex reveals essential interactions between snake alpha-neurotoxins and nicotinic receptors." EMBO J **24**(8): 1512-22.

Brejc, K., *et al.* (2001). "Crystal structure of an ACh-binding protein reveals the ligand-binding domain of nicotinic receptors." Nature **411**(6835): 269-76.

Cascio, M. (2004). "Structure and function of the glycine receptor and related nicotinicoid receptors." J Biol Chem **279**(19): 19383-6.

Celie, P. H., *et al.* (2004). "Nicotine and carbamylcholine binding to nicotinic acetylcholine receptors as studied in AChBP crystal structures." Neuron **41**(6): 907-14.
Cheng, J., *et al.* (2009). "Homology modeling of human alpha1beta2gamma2 and house fly beta3 GABA receptor channels and Surflex-docking of fipronil." J Mol Model.
Cheng, X., *et al.* (2007). "Nanosecond-timescale conformational dynamics of the human alpha7 nicotinic acetylcholine receptor." Biophys J **93**(8): 2622-34.
Corringer, P. J., *et al.* (2000). "Nicotinic receptors at the amino acid level." Annu Rev Pharmacol Toxicol **40**: 431-58.
Dellisanti, C. D., *et al.* (2007). "Crystal structure of the extracellular domain of nAChR alpha1 bound to alpha-bungarotoxin at 1.94 A resolution." Nat Neurosci **10**(8): 953-62.
Dennis, M., *et al.* (1988). "Amino acids of the Torpedo marmorata acetylcholine receptor alpha subunit labeled by a photoaffinity ligand for the acetylcholine binding site." Biochemistry **27**(7): 2346-57.
Dutertre, S. and R. J. Lewis (2006). "Toxin insights into nicotinic acetylcholine receptors." Biochem Pharmacol **72**(6): 661-70.
Dutertre, S., *et al.* (2004). "Determination of alpha-conotoxin binding modes on neuronal nicotinic acetylcholine receptors." J Mol Recognit **17**(4): 339-47.
Edelstein, S. J., *et al.* (1996). "A kinetic mechanism for nicotinic acetylcholine receptors based on multiple allosteric transitions." Biol Cybern **75**(5): 361-79.
Esnouf, R. M. (1997). "An extensively modified version of MolScript that includes greatly enhanced coloring capabilities." J Mol Graph Model **15**(2): 132-4, 112-3.
Farrant, M. and Z. Nusser (2005). "Variations on an inhibitory theme: phasic and tonic activation of GABA(A) receptors." Nat Rev Neurosci **6**(3): 215-29.
Forrest, L. R. and M. S. Sansom (2000). "Membrane simulations: bigger and better?" Curr Opin Struct Biol **10**(2): 174-81.
Gabb, H. A., *et al.* (1997). "Modelling protein docking using shape complementarity, electrostatics and biochemical information." J Mol Biol **272**(1): 106-20.
Ghijsen, W. E. and A. G. Leenders (2005). "Differential signaling in presynaptic neurotransmitter release." Cell Mol Life Sci **62**(9): 937-54.
Goodsell, D. S. (2005). "Representing structural information with RasMol." Curr Protoc Bioinformatics **Chapter 5**: Unit 5 4.
Goodsell, D. S., *et al.* (1996). "Automated docking of flexible ligands: applications of AutoDock." J Mol Recognit **9**(1): 1-5.
Groebe, D. R. and S. N. Abramson (1995). "Lophotoxin is a slow binding irreversible inhibitor of nicotinic acetylcholine receptors." J Biol Chem **270**(1): 281-6.
Grosman, C., *et al.* (2000). "The extracellular linker of muscle acetylcholine receptor channels is a gating control element." J Gen Physiol **116**(3): 327-40.
Grosman, C., *et al.* (2000). "Mapping the conformational wave of acetylcholine receptor channel gating." Nature **403**(6771): 773-6.
Haddadian, E. J., *et al.* (2008). "In silico models for the human alpha4beta2 nicotinic acetylcholine receptor." J Phys Chem B **112**(44): 13981-90.
Harel, M., *et al.* (2001). "The binding site of acetylcholine receptor as visualized in the X-Ray structure of a complex between alpha-bungarotoxin and a mimotope peptide." Neuron **32**(2): 265-75.
Hogg, R. C. and D. Bertrand (2007). "Partial agonists as therapeutic agents at neuronal nicotinic acetylcholine receptors." Biochem Pharmacol **73**(4): 459-68.
Holladay, M. W., *et al.* (1997). "Neuronal nicotinic acetylcholine receptors as targets for drug discovery." J Med Chem **40**(26): 4169-94.

Holm, L. and J. Park (2000). "DaliLite workbench for protein structure comparison." Bioinformatics **16**(6): 566-7.

Innis, C. A., *et al.* (2000). "Evolutionary trace analysis of TGF-beta and related growth factors: implications for site-directed mutagenesis." Protein Eng **13**(12): 839-47.

Itier, V. and D. Bertrand (2001). "Neuronal nicotinic receptors: from protein structure to function." FEBS Lett **504**(3): 118-25.

Jackson, M. B. (1989). "Perfection of a synaptic receptor: kinetics and energetics of the acetylcholine receptor." Proc Natl Acad Sci U S A **86**(7): 2199-203.

Janes, R. W. (2003). "Nicotinic acetylcholine receptors: alpha-conotoxins as templates for rational drug design." Biochem Soc Trans **31**(Pt 3): 634-6.

Janes, R. W. (2005). "alpha-Conotoxins as selective probes for nicotinic acetylcholine receptor subclasses." Curr Opin Pharmacol **5**(3): 280-92.

Jensen, A. A., *et al.* (2005). "Neuronal nicotinic acetylcholine receptors: structural revelations, target identifications, and therapeutic inspirations." J Med Chem **48**(15): 4705-45.

Jones, S. and J. M. Thornton (1995). "Protein-protein interactions: a review of protein dimer structures." Prog Biophys Mol Biol **63**(1): 31-65.

Kandt, C., *et al.* (2007). "Setting up and running molecular dynamics simulations of membrane proteins." Methods **41**(4): 475-88.

Kandt, C., *et al.* (2005). "Water dynamics simulation as a tool for probing proton transfer pathways in a heptahelical membrane protein." Proteins **58**(3): 528-37.

Kaplan, W. and T. G. Littlejohn (2001). "Swiss-PDB Viewer (Deep View)." Brief Bioinform **2**(2): 195-7.

Karlin, A. (2002). "Emerging structure of the nicotinic acetylcholine receptors." Nat Rev Neurosci **3**(2): 102-14.

Kash, T. L., *et al.* (2004). "Structural elements involved in activation of the gamma-aminobutyric acid type A (GABAA) receptor." Biochem Soc Trans **32**(Pt3): 540-6.

Katchalski-Katzir, E., *et al.* (1992). "Molecular surface recognition: determination of geometric fit between proteins and their ligands by correlation techniques." Proc Natl Acad Sci U S A **89**(6): 2195-9.

Khalili-Araghi, F., *et al.* (2009). "Molecular dynamics simulations of membrane channels and transporters." Curr Opin Struct Biol **19**(2): 128-37.

Konstantakaki, M., *et al.* (2007). "Docking of alpha-cobratoxin suggests a basal conformation of the nicotinic receptor." Biochem Biophys Res Commun **359**(3): 413-8.

Konstantakaki, M., *et al.* (2007). "Molecular modeling of the complex between Torpedo acetylcholine receptor and anti-MIR Fab198." Biochem Biophys Res Commun **356**(3): 569-75.

Konstantakaki, M., *et al.* (2008). "Model of the extracellular domain of the human alpha7 nAChR based on the crystal structure of the mouse alpha1 nAChR extracellular domain." J Mol Graph Model **26**(8): 1333-7.

Kutzner, C., *et al.* (2007). "Speeding up parallel GROMACS on high-latency networks." J Comput Chem **28**(12): 2075-84.

Laskowski, R. A., *et al.* (1993). "Main-chain bond lengths and bond angles in protein structures." J Mol Biol **231**(4): 1049-67.

Law, R. J., *et al.* (2000). "Structure and dynamics of the pore-lining helix of the nicotinic receptor: MD simulations in water, lipid bilayers, and transbilayer bundles." Proteins **39**(1): 47-55.

Le Novere, N. and J. P. Changeux (1995). "Molecular evolution of the nicotinic acetylcholine receptor: an example of multigene family in excitable cells." J Mol Evol **40**(2): 155-72.

Le Novere, N. and J. P. Changeux (2001). "LGICdb: the ligand-gated ion channel database." Nucleic Acids Res **29**(1): 294-5.

Le Novere, N. and J. P. Changeux (2001). "The Ligand Gated Ion Channel database: an example of a sequence database in neuroscience." Philos Trans R Soc Lond B Biol Sci **356**(1412): 1121-30.

Le Novere, N., *et al.* (1999). "Improved secondary structure predictions for a nicotinic receptor subunit: incorporation of solvent accessibility and experimental data into a two-dimensional representation." Biophys J **76**(5): 2329-45.

Leonard, S. and D. Bertrand (2001). "Neuronal nicotinic receptors: from structure to function." Nicotine Tob Res **3**(3): 203-23.

Lewis, R. J. and M. L. Garcia (2003). "Therapeutic potential of venom peptides." Nat Rev Drug Discov **2**(10): 790-802.

Lichtarge, O., *et al.* (1996). "An evolutionary trace method defines binding surfaces common to protein families." J Mol Biol **257**(2): 342-58.

Lichtarge, O. and M. E. Sowa (2002). "Evolutionary predictions of binding surfaces and interactions." Curr Opin Struct Biol **12**(1): 21-7.

Liu, X., *et al.* (2008). "Mechanics of channel gating of the nicotinic acetylcholine receptor." PLoS Comput Biol **4**(1): e19.

Lloyd, G. K. and M. Williams (2000). "Neuronal nicotinic acetylcholine receptors as novel drug targets." J Pharmacol Exp Ther **292**(2): 461-7.

Lombard, V., *et al.* (2002). "EMBL-Align: a new public nucleotide and amino acid multiple sequence alignment database." Bioinformatics **18**(5): 763-4.

MacDermott, A. B., *et al.* (1999). "Presynaptic ionotropic receptors and the control of transmitter release." Annu Rev Neurosci **22**: 443-85.

McGuffin, L. J., *et al.* (2000). "The PSIPRED protein structure prediction server." Bioinformatics **16**(4): 404-5.

McGuffin, L. J. and D. T. Jones (2003). "Improvement of the GenTHREADER method for genomic fold recognition." Bioinformatics **19**(7): 874-81.

Morris, A. L., *et al.* (1992). "Stereochemical quality of protein structure coordinates." Proteins **12**(4): 345-64.

Morris, G. M., *et al.* (1996). "Distributed automated docking of flexible ligands to proteins: parallel applications of AutoDock 2.4." J Comput Aided Mol Des **10**(4): 293-304.

Morris, G. M., *et al.* (2009). "AutoDock4 and AutoDockTools4: Automated docking with selective receptor flexibility." J Comput Chem.

Morris, G. M., *et al.* (2008). "Using AutoDock for ligand-receptor docking." Curr Protoc Bioinformatics **Chapter 8**: Unit 8 14.

Nasiripourdori, A., *et al.* (2009). "Binding of long-chain alpha-neurotoxin would stabilize the resting state of nAChR: a comparative study with alpha-conotoxin." Theor Biol Med Model **6**: 3.

Nicke, A., *et al.* (2003). "Alpha-conotoxins EpI and AuIB switch subtype selectivity and activity in native versus recombinant nicotinic acetylcholine receptors." FEBS Lett **554**(1-2): 219-23.

Nicke, A., *et al.* (2004). "Alpha-conotoxins as tools for the elucidation of structure and function of neuronal nicotinic acetylcholine receptor subtypes." Eur J Biochem **271**(12): 2305-19.

Nowak, M. W., *et al.* (1995). "Nicotinic receptor binding site probed with unnatural amino acid incorporation in intact cells." Science **268**(5209): 439-42.

Opella, S. J., *et al.* (1999). "Structures of the M2 channel-lining segments from nicotinic acetylcholine and NMDA receptors by NMR spectroscopy." Nat Struct Biol **6**(4): 374-9.

Orengo, C. A., *et al.* (1999). "Analysis and assessment of ab initio three-dimensional prediction, secondary structure, and contacts prediction." Proteins **Suppl 3**: 149-70.

Osterberg, F., *et al.* (2002). "Automated docking to multiple target structures: incorporation of protein mobility and structural water heterogeneity in AutoDock." Proteins **46**(1): 34-40.

Parthiban, M., *et al.* (2009). "Molecular modeling of human pentameric alpha(7) neuronal nicotinic acetylcholine receptor and its interaction with its agonist and competitive antagonist." J Biomol Struct Dyn **26**(5): 535-47.

Prince, R. J. and S. M. Sine (1999). "Acetylcholine and epibatidine binding to muscle acetylcholine receptors distinguish between concerted and uncoupled models." J Biol Chem **274**(28): 19623-9.

Quick, M. W. and R. A. Lester (2002). "Desensitization of neuronal nicotinic receptors." J Neurobiol **53**(4): 457-78.

Retief, J. D. (2000). "Phylogenetic analysis using PHYLIP." Methods Mol Biol **132**: 243-58.

Revah, F., *et al.* (1991). "Mutations in the channel domain alter desensitization of a neuronal nicotinic receptor." Nature **353**(6347): 846-9.

Russell, R. B., *et al.* (1997). "Recognition of analogous and homologous protein folds: analysis of sequence and structure conservation." J Mol Biol **269**(3): 423-39.

Sali, A. and T. L. Blundell (1993). "Comparative protein modelling by satisfaction of spatial restraints." J Mol Biol **234**(3): 779-815.

Salvaterra, P. M. and W. J. Moore (1973). "Binding of (125I)-alpha bungarotoxin to particulate fractions of rat and guinea pig brain." Biochem Biophys Res Commun **55**(4): 1311-8.

Sansom, M. S., *et al.* (1998). "Modelling and simulation of ion channels: applications to the nicotinic acetylcholine receptor." J Struct Biol **121**(2): 246-62.

Sansom, M. S., *et al.* (2002). "Water in ion channels and pores--simulation studies." Novartis Found Symp **245**: 66-78; discussion 79-83, 165-8.

Sayle, R. A. and E. J. Milner-White (1995). "RASMOL: biomolecular graphics for all." Trends Biochem Sci **20**(9): 374.

Schapira, M., *et al.* (2002). "Structural model of nicotinic acetylcholine receptor isotypes bound to acetylcholine and nicotine." BMC Struct Biol **2**: 1.

Schuttelkopf, A. W. and D. M. van Aalten (2004). "PRODRG: a tool for high-throughput crystallography of protein-ligand complexes." Acta Crystallogr D Biol Crystallogr **60**(Pt 8): 1355-63.

Sgrignani, J., *et al.* (2009). "Insights into docking and scoring neuronal alpha4beta2 nicotinic receptor agonists using molecular dynamics simulations and QM/MM calculations." J Comput Chem.

Shen, J. X. and J. L. Yakel (2009). "Nicotinic acetylcholine receptor-mediated calcium signaling in the nervous system." Acta Pharmacol Sin **30**(6): 673-80.

Smit, A. B., *et al.* (2001). "A glia-derived acetylcholine-binding protein that modulates synaptic transmission." Nature **411**(6835): 261-8.

Sobolev, V., *et al.* (1999). "Automated analysis of interatomic contacts in proteins." Bioinformatics **15**(4): 327-32.

Soriano, E., *et al.* (2009). "Computational analysis of the binding ability of heterocyclic and conformationally constrained epibatidine analogs in the neuronal nicotinic acetylcholine receptor." Mol Divers.

Stoesser, G., *et al.* (2002). "The EMBL Nucleotide Sequence Database." Nucleic Acids Res **30**(1): 21-6.

Tang, P., *et al.* (2002). "NMR structures of the second transmembrane domain of the human glycine receptor alpha(1) subunit: model of pore architecture and channel gating." Biophys J **83**(1): 252-62.

Tang, P. A., *et al.* (2009). "Molecular characterization of two nicotinic acetylcholine receptor subunits from Liposcelis bostrychophila Badonnel (Psocoptera: Liposcelididae)." Arch Insect Biochem Physiol.

Thompson, J. D., *et al.* (2002). "Multiple sequence alignment using ClustalW and ClustalX." Curr Protoc Bioinformatics **Chapter 2**: Unit 2 3.

Tuppo, E. E. and H. R. Arias (2005). "The role of inflammation in Alzheimer's disease." Int J Biochem Cell Biol **37**(2): 289-305.

Unwin, N. (2005). "Refined structure of the nicotinic acetylcholine receptor at 4A resolution." J Mol Biol **346**(4): 967-89.

Unwin, N., *et al.* (2002). "Activation of the nicotinic acetylcholine receptor involves a switch in conformation of the alpha subunits." J Mol Biol **319**(5): 1165-76.

Van Der Spoel, D., *et al.* (2005). "GROMACS: fast, flexible, and free." J Comput Chem **26**(16): 1701-18.

Vriend, G. (1990). "WHAT IF: a molecular modeling and drug design program." J Mol Graph **8**(1): 52-6, 29.

Wallace, A. C., *et al.* (1995). "LIGPLOT: a program to generate schematic diagrams of protein-ligand interactions." Protein Eng **8**(2): 127-34.

Ward, R. M., *et al.* (2009). "Evolutionary Trace Annotation Server: automated enzyme function prediction in protein structures using 3D templates." Bioinformatics **25**(11): 1426-7.

Willard, L., *et al.* (2003). "VADAR: a web server for quantitative evaluation of protein structure quality." Nucleic Acids Res **31**(13): 3316-9.

Yogeeswari, P., *et al.* (2006). "Epibatidine and its analogues as nicotinic acetylcholine receptor agonist: an update." Nat Prod Res **20**(5): 497-505.

Zingsheim, H. P., *et al.* (1982). "Direct structural localization of two toxin-recognition sites on an ACh receptor protein." Nature **299**(5878): 81-4.

Printed in Great Britain
by Amazon

45697972R00072